RESEARCH STRATEGIES IN HUMAN COMMUNICATION DISORDERS

RESEARCH STRATEGIES IN HUMAN COMMUNICATION DISORDERS

DONALD G. DOEHRING, PH.D.

School of Human Communication Disorders,
McGill University
Montreal, Canada

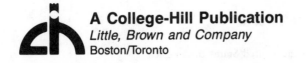

A College-Hill Publication
Little, Brown and Company
Boston/Toronto

College-Hill Press
A Division of
Little, Brown and Company (Inc.)
34 Beacon Street
Boston, Massachusetts 02108

Library of Congress Cataloging in Publication Data
Main entry under title:

Doehring, Donald G.
    Research strategies in human communication disorders / Donald G.
    Doehring.
        p.   cm.
    "A College-Hill publication."
    Includes bibliographies and index.
    1. Communicative disorders—Research—Methodology. I. Title.
    [DNLM: 1. Communicative Disorders. 2. Research Design. WL 340
    D649]
    RC429.D64 1988
    616.85′5—dc19
    DNLM/DLC   88–12759
                                                                    CIP

ISBN 0-316-18900-6

Printed in the United States of America

CONTENTS

To Eileen

PREFACE

This book is intended for anyone, including students, teachers, practitioners, and researchers, interested in research in human communication disorders. Its purpose is to describe how research is actually done. Examples of research in human communication disorders are given throughout the book, and readers are referred to journals to find other examples.

There is equal emphasis on research methods and research strategies. The major part of the book is devoted to a systematic description of planning, carrying out, analyzing, and interpreting research. Basic concepts and principles are presented in a step-by-step manner. Both standard group designs and other approaches are described. The most detailed attention is given to research design and statistical analysis, since these are the aspects of human communication disorders research that are most difficult to learn and to apply.

The aim is to describe the purpose and the function of each aspect of research rather than to give complete technical details. Readers who are familiar with research methods and statistical analysis can see how the methods and techniques are applied to human communication disorders research. Readers who require additional information are referred to texts containing more detailed explanations. Review questions and exercises are included to help in understanding special terms, concepts, and methods.

The importance of knowing how to evaluate the strengths and weaknesses of different research approaches is emphasized. As each research event is described, there is a discussion of strategies for dealing with practical limitations. The final chapter is devoted to a general discussion of the strategies required for a well-integrated approach to research in human communication disorders.

Advice about how to critically evaluate research, conduct research, and write research reports is given in the appendices.

It is hoped this book will inspire readers to join the quest for useful knowledge about human communication disorders.

ACKNOWLEDGMENTS

I wish to thank Daniel Ling, my friend and editor, for guidance and critical comments. Others who made valuable suggestions include my colleagues Elizabeth Cole, Martha Crago, Tanya Gallagher, and James McNutt. Donald Polkinghorne helped me to understand the application of nonstandard research approaches. Dean Richard Cruess of the McGill Faculty of Medicine has unfailingly supported my efforts to advance research in human communication disorders. I am greatly indebted to my mentor, Hallowell Davis, and to my late colleague and friend, Bonnie Bryans, for whatever success I have had in expressing my ideas about research in a clear and logical manner.

Introduction

Human communication disorders (HCDs) are speaking and listening difficulties that impair communication. They range from defective speech and impaired hearing to deficiencies in understanding and expressing communicative intentions. There are many persons with HCDs. They occur in both children and adults, and can be present at birth or acquired later in life.

The goal of HCD research is to obtain useful knowledge. Many different kinds of knowledge can be useful. An example of useful knowledge that might be obtained about one particular HCD will illustrate this.

AN EXAMPLE OF RESEARCH IN HUMAN COMMUNICATION DISORDERS

Children who make certain errors of omission, distortion, or substitution of speech sounds have communication disorders called *articulation disorders* or *phonological disorders*. Knowledge obtained by research on the following topics could prove useful for helping children with these disorders.

1

Incidence of Disorders

Researchers could carry out survey research to determine how frequently articulation/phonological disorders occur. This information would help in the planning of effective programs for dealing with these disorders.

Self-Limiting Nature of Disorders

Research aimed at determining whether some or all children with articulation/phonological disorders outgrow them without any special help could also provide very useful information for program planning.

Assessment of Disorders

Procedures for reliable assessment of the disorders could be developed through research. Such procedures would be needed for research on the incidence and the self-limiting nature of the disorders.

Effects of Intervention

Research that evaluates the effectiveness of procedures for dealing with articulation/phonological disorders would provide still another type of very useful information for program planning.

Associated Deficits

Researchers could determine what other deficits might be present in children with these disorders. Deficits that might be associated with articulation/phonological disorders include deficiencies in the physical structures (mouth, throat, respiratory system) involved in speech, deficiencies of sensory systems (touch, position) involved in speech, deficiencies in other types of movement (e.g., finger movements), deficiencies in the perception as well as the production of speech sounds, and deficiencies in higher-level language abilities. Knowledge about associated deficits could be of direct or indirect help in planning more effective ways of helping children with these problems.

Causes of Disorders

Research on associated deficits could indicate the extent to which articulation/phonological disorders might be the result of structural abnormalities, sensory deficits, general movement disorders, perceptual disorders, or language disorders. Even if no deficits of these types were found, there might be subtle deficiencies in the brain mechanisms that coordinate speech movements. Information about such associated deficits could be used in further research into the causes of these disorders. It would be necessary to determine the role played by the "organic factors" involved in associated deficits, and also the role played by experience. The researchers would have to determine the extent to which organic and experiential factors might operate jointly to cause articulation/phonological disorders. Research into the causes of disorders is especially difficult, but any information obtained by research would be very important for planning the most effective ways of helping children with these disorders.

Unitary Nature of Disorders

Research concerned with the effects of training, associated deficits, and possible causes should provide some suggestion as to whether there is a single type of articulation/phonological disorder with a single cause, a single pattern of associated deficit, and a common response to training. If there does not appear to be a unitary disorder, research could be carried out to determine the number and types of different articulation/phonological disorders. This information could help in the planning of programs that would be much more effective for individual children.

Evaluation of Different Methods of Intervention

Research could be carried out to evaluate procedures for dealing with the articulation/phonological disorders. The procedures evaluated could include different training methods and different methods for counseling the child and the child's parents and teachers. If there is not a unitary disorder, different procedures might prove appropriate for different types of disorder. An important aspect of this type of research would be the choice of methods to be compared. All of the information available from previous research, from theories of articulation/phonological disorders, and from practitioners' experience would be useful in choosing the methods most likely to be effective.

Effects on Communication

It would also be important to determine the effects of articulation/phonological disorders on communication. If the disorders do not impede communication and are self-limiting, formal programs for helping children with these disorders might not be needed. Factors other than poor speech that might impede communication could be the reactions of others during communicative interactions, and the attitudes of parents and teachers toward speech defects. Information about these effects of articulation/phonological disorders could be very useful. For example, one way to deal with the disorders might be to change the way others react to them.

Effects on Communication Development

If articulation/phonological disorders do impede communication, it would be necessary to determine whether children with these disorders have difficulty in the development of skills for interactive communication. If so, it would be important to deal with the disorders as soon as possible, even if the children would eventually grow out of them.

As this example indicates, many different kinds of useful knowledge can be obtained by research even when only one specific type of HCD is considered. The exact type of research that will provide useful knowledge depends on the type of disorder. Less extensive programs of research might be required for some disorders, and more extensive programs might be required for others.

THE USES OF KNOWLEDGE OBTAINED BY RESEARCH

Some knowledge obtained by research might be directly applied. More effective training methods and improved speech aids and hearing aids could be adopted immediately, providing that enough knowledge about them was obtained by research.

Other knowledge obtained by research could be applied through changes in practice. In the example of articulation/phonological disorders, knowledge about the incidence and the self-limiting nature of disorders and about the effectiveness of treatment could help in the planning of programs for dealing with the disorders.

An indirect effect of research would be to change theories. Theories concerning articulation/phonological disorders that might be changed by research include theories about associated deficits, causes, and different types of disorders, as well as theories about how best to eliminate disorders and theories about the effects of disorders on communication. Some of these theories could be directly applied to practice and others would need to be modified on the basis of further research before they could be applied.

The most indirect effect of research would be to suggest further research. Further research could provide additional information about the same problem, or it could advance to a further stage of inquiry. For example, knowledge about deficits associated with articulation/phonological disorders might lead to research into the causes of the disorders, and research on causality might lead to research on methods for dealing with the disorders. Further research would be continued until the knowledge obtained could be applied to theories or practice.

THE NATURE OF KNOWLEDGE OBTAINED BY RESEARCH

HCD research is not usually aimed at the discovery of absolute truth or universal scientific laws. The knowledge obtained is provisional. The practical needs for dealing with HCDs require that knowledge obtained by research be put to use whenever possible. The kinds of social and cultural processes involved in human communication continue to evolve.

The distinction between provisional knowledge and universal scientific laws is important. Research methods designed for the discovery of universal scientific laws may not always be appropriate for HCD research.

THE EVALUATION OF KNOWLEDGE OBTAINED BY RESEARCH

Provisional knowledge about human communication disorders is obtained by a variety of research methods. Before the knowledge can be used, it must be evaluated by experts who are familiar with both the methods and the subject matter of the research. A common form of evaluation is the review by experts of research reports submitted for publication in professional journals. This type of *peer evaluation* is the standard procedure for establishing the acceptability of knowledge obtained by research. Because the knowledge is provisional, later research may provide supplementary or contradictory knowledge.

It is important to understand that knowledge obtained by HCD research is not necessarily permanent or infallible. Knowledge about HCDs is obtained by the astute application of available methods, with peer evaluation of the results.

THE NEED FOR KNOWLEDGE OBTAINED BY RESEARCH

Some kinds of provisional knowledge about HCDs are derived from practical experience or theoretical speculation. However, when HCDs are at all complex and variable, research may be necessary to untangle the complexities and account for the sources of variability. Provisional knowledge based on practical experience or intuitive speculation is less likely to be useful for helping persons with HCDs. Careful research is the best way to obtain information about such matters as the incidence of disorders, the causes of disorders, the characteristics of disorders, the effectiveness of treatments, and the effects of disorders on communication. Where research has not yet obtained the desired information, knowledge derived from practical experience and theoretical speculation must be used.

RESEARCH AND THEORY

Knowledge obtained by research may provide useful information for theories of HCDs. Where knowledge from HCD research and from theories and research concerning normal human communication is not sufficient, theories may also be based in part on practical knowledge about HCDs. Then theorists must fill any remaining gaps in knowledge with their own speculations. An important function of research is to provide theorists with as much peer-evaluated knowledge as possible.

Theories integrate information from all sources into useful explanations of HCDs. The theory is the means for summing up current knowledge. Well-organized theories can be systematically revised on the basis of information obtained by research.

HCD theories are usually constructed by researchers or practitioners, and there can be many different theories. As HCD theories evolve, they become more applicable to practice, thus closing the gap between theory and practice. The knowledge obtained by research can help theories evolve in this direction.

RESEARCH AND PRACTICE

In deciding how best to deal with HCDs such as articulation/phonological disorders, practitioners use whatever knowledge is available from theories, research, and practical experience. When knowledge is incomplete, they have to make the most informed guesses possible. More guesswork is required for some disorders than for others. There is a similarity between theory and practice in this respect.

The knowledge obtained by research can reduce the guesswork in practice either by direct application or by contributing to the theories that practitioners use. Research can be of most help where there is less knowledge and more guesswork. In such cases, the knowledge obtained by research would most likely be applied to HCD theories.

THE CHALLENGE OF HCD RESEARCH

The challenge for HCD researchers is to make the best use of available methods to obtain useful knowledge. The task is not simple, since many different kinds of knowledge are necessary. HCD researchers must attempt to supply knowledge wherever it is lacking. In addition to practical applications, research may be needed to improve theories of HCDs or to provide a basis for further research.

HCD researchers do not work in isolated laboratories, carefully applying precise methods for discovering universal laws. They determine what knowledge about HCDs is needed and then try to obtain it as best they can. Their efforts are evaluated by experts who decide whether the knowledge is acceptable. Then the knowledge may be directly or indirectly put to the practical use of helping the communicatively disordered.

Difficult though it may be, HCD research offers researchers the opportunity to make important contributions to society. The stakes are high. Practitioners help those with whom they work, whereas research can provide information that will help everyone who has an HCD.

RESEARCH METHODS AND RESEARCH STRATEGIES

Researchers must use established methods in order that their findings will be accepted as valid contributions to knowledge. However, expert researchers, like expert practitioners, do not mechanically apply methods. Each research problem, like each person with an HCD, is unique. Researchers have to adapt available methods to fit each problem. To do so, they must be familiar with current methods and on the lookout for better ones. The term *research strategy* provides an appropriate description of the activities of HCD researchers.

PLAN OF THIS BOOK

This book describes how research methods and strategies are applied to obtain useful knowledge about HCDs. Following the discussion of research, theory, and practice in this chapter, the sequence of events in research is described in Chapter 2, and the different types of HCD research are described in Chapter 3. Then the details of designing, carrying out, analyzing, and interpreting research are given in Chapters 4 to 16. Research strategies are discussed in the final chapter. Practical advice about how to read and evaluate research reports, how to do research, and how to prepare research reports is given in the appendices.

Throughout the book there is an emphasis on actual examples of HCD research. The best way to learn about HCD research is to understand the basic principles and techniques, find examples of their application by researchers, and then begin to apply them.

ADDITIONAL INFORMATION

Additional information about the special nature of HCD research is given in books by Hegde (1987), McReynolds and Kearns (1983), Shearer (1982), Silverman (1977), and Ventry and Schiavetti (1980).

REVIEW QUESTIONS

1. Referring to the example of different types of research on articulation/phonological disorders, describe the kinds of useful knowledge that might be obtained by research on another HCD such as conductive hearing loss or aphasia.
2. Describe the relationship between research, theory, and practice.
3. Why is the term *research strategy* used in connection with HCD research?

The Sequence of Events in Research

This chapter describes the events involved in HCD research and how they are reported in published studies. The sequence of events is simple: Researchers identify an important gap in knowledge concerning HCDs, decide on a specific purpose, make a plan for achieving the purpose, and then collect, analyze, and interpret the evidence. Research is a well-organized exploration.

In published research reports, the events are reported in their order of occurrence, as shown in Table 2–1:

TABLE 2–1.
Order of Occurrence of Research Events in Research Reports.

Research Events	Research Reports
PROBLEM (Gap in knowledge about HCDs)	INTRODUCTION
PURPOSE (Specific aspects to be studied	INTRODUCTION
DESIGN (Plan for achieving the purpose)	INTRODUCTION, METHOD
PROCEDURE (Operations for carrying out plan)	METHOD
ANALYSIS (Organization of findings)	METHOD, RESULTS
INTERPRETATION (Evaluating findings)	DISCUSSION

Each of the events is essential and has its own special importance. The research events will be described in relation to the sections of published research reports.

THE PROBLEM

Finding the Problem

Students who are beginning research may learn about a challenging problem from their study of the literature, or from a researcher, teacher, or clinical supervisor. They may become interested in a particular HCD and then look for a gap in knowledge concerning that HCD through reading and consulting experts. Or, they may join a research team that is investigating a particular problem.

Practitioners may become interested in research because they have identified an important gap in knowledge through their clinical work. Then they might seek the collaboration of researchers to plan and carry out research that will reduce the gap.

Experienced researchers often identify a problem through their own previous research. Most gaps in knowledge are not filled by a single study, but require a series of related studies. One of the most important research skills is to decide exactly what problem to investigate at each stage in a series of studies.

Importance of the Problem

Some research efforts contribute small amounts and others, large amounts of knowledge. Everyone is familiar with scientists who stumble on important discoveries by accident. We cannot predict which studies will turn out to be the most important. Both chance and the intuition of the researcher play a part. However, the better informed and the more thoughtful the researcher in selecting the problem, the more likely it is to be important.

Specifying the Problem

Once a gap in knowledge is found, the researcher has to look for previous research and theories that confirm the existence of the gap and define it more precisely. This is done by reading relevant books and journals and consulting experts. A great deal of reading and consultation may be needed. The most recent research and theories can be found by reading current issues and consulting annual indexes of relevant journals, writing to leading researchers, and attending research conferences. Computer searches of the literature are also helpful. Where there has not been a thorough search for previous studies on the topic, the knowledge obtained by research may be of little value. There may be repetition of studies that have already been done, or failure to take into consideration important factors discovered by previous researchers.

Statement of the Problem in Research Reports

The gap in knowledge studied by the researcher is described in the first section of the research report. The problem is usually introduced by a discussion of theories and research relating to the gap in knowledge. This defines the general problem area. Then research and theory directly related to the problem are described in more detail, and the gap in knowledge is stated in more specific terms.

The background information and the statement of the problem establish the importance of the research. The editors and reviewers of the journal serve as a jury of peers. They will not accept the research report for publication if they decide that the gap in knowledge has not been adequately defined or the problem is not important. The researcher not only has to find an important problem, but present sufficient background information within a page or two to demonstrate its importance. Problems are important to the extent that knowledge obtained about them will directly or indirectly be of benefit to persons with HCDs.

Examples of Important Problems

There are many important gaps in knowledge about HCDs, such as the most effective methods for developing language in children with congenital hearing impairment, the exact characteristics of developmental central auditory disorders and language disorders, and the causes of stuttering and articulation/phonological disorders. Such problems are too large to be dealt with by a single research study.

Published studies represent realistic attempts to make progress by obtaining information about selected aspects of important problems. Examples of actual gaps in knowledge defined as research problems by HCD researchers can be seen in the first six research reports in the June 1987 issue of the *Journal of Speech and Hearing Research* (JSHR):

1. Evaluation of methods for overcoming the effects of tinnitus (ringing in the ears)
2. Evaluation of methods for auditory training of adults with acquired sensorineural loss

3. Determination of the normal limits of ear drum and acoustic reflex responses

4. Description of the tongue movements of children with articulation disorders

5. Assessment of the story-telling skills of children with language disorders

6. Determination of how patients with voice disorders control their vocal muscles.

All of these problems were judged important enough for publication in JSHR. Some involved direct attempts to close gaps in knowledge, whereas others were less direct. Overcoming tinnitus and auditory training of the hearing impaired are direct attempts to obtain information for helping persons with HCDs. Measurements of ear drum and acoustic reflex responses, tongue movements, story-telling skills, and vocal muscle control can lead to better ways of assessing and treating HCDs.

A careful reading of the introductory sections of the six research reports will indicate how the researchers describe the background of the problems. The practical importance is not always spelled out, as it is assumed that readers have some previous knowledge of the topic.

THE PURPOSE

After identifying the problem, researchers have to plan a study that will reduce the gap in knowledge. The plan is related to the problem by a statement of the specific purpose of the research. Then a study is designed to accomplish the purpose. Planning continues until a study has been designed that fits the purpose and provides acceptable evidence. If a design that will accomplish the purpose cannot be found, the purpose must be modified to fit the available designs.

The Statement of Purpose

The purpose specifies the aspect of the problem that will be investigated. It indicates how much of the gap in knowledge will be reduced and defines the task of research design.

In published HCD research reports, the purpose of the study is usually stated toward the end of the introductory section, sometimes indirectly. The following statements of purpose are taken from the first six reports in the June 1987 issue of JSHR:

1. This paper is concerned with specification of the characteristics of external stimuli that mask tinnitus and with whether the tinnitus is

masked centrally (i.e., retrocochlearly) or peripherally (i.e., in the cochlea) (Penner, 1987, p. 147).

2. The goals of the present study were to determine (a) whether performance on tasks of speech recognition would improve in response to training, . . . and (d) whether any measured improvements would be retained after training ended (Rubenstein & Boothroyd, 1987, p. 153).

3. Accordingly, the purpose of the present study was to provide a preliminary data base of acoustic-immitance measures in normal ears (Wiley, Oviatt, & Block, 1987, p. 161).

4. It is suggested that a detailed analysis of lingual-contact data together with an auditory-based analysis will provide an objective empirically based framework for a more adequate categorization of the disorders (Hardcastle, Barry, & Clark, 1987, p. 172).

5. The present investigation will extend the findings by previous investigators by determining if the ability to access any of the proposed levels (i.e., macrolevel, microlevel, social) during narrative discourse will distinguish language-disordered children from children with normal language ability (Liles, 1987, p. 186).

6. Because the speech tasks required different degrees of dynamic and precise vocal fold control, the purpose was to improve our understanding of the voluntary laryngeal movement disorders in SD [spastic dysphonia] (Ludlow & Connor, 1987, p. 198).

These statements of purpose tend to be very specific in comparison with the descriptions of the problem listed in the previous section.

THE DESIGN

Researchers have to plan research that will provide the information specified by the statement of purpose. The plan involves the selection of an appropriate research design. A number of different kinds of research designs are available for use. To plan, understand, and evaluate HCD research it is necessary to be familiar with the most commonly used designs. Research designs are briefly described here to indicate their function in the sequence of research events. A detailed description of research designs is given in Chapters 4 to 8.

The most common designs provide information about one or more groups, using methods developed for psychological research. Information about the characteristics of HCDs can be obtained by comparing groups with HCDs to groups without HCDs, by comparing groups with different types of HCDs, or by analyzing relevant characteristics of a single group. Information about the effectiveness of methods for helping persons with

HCDs can be obtained by assessing groups with HCDs before and after the methods have been applied. The information provided by group studies is usually evaluated by statistical analyses which estimate the probability that the observed effects would occur in persons with that type of HCD.

Groups can also be studied by methods that do not lead to probability estimates. Some of these methods involve quantitative and others, qualitative descriptions of groups. Group descriptive designs involve quantitative descriptions of the characteristics of a population, with no comparisons between groups or between experimental conditions.

Information about the characteristics of HCDs or the effects of treatment can also be obtained by intensive study of individuals with HCDs. When studying stable individual characteristics, quantitative descriptions of individuals may be adequate. A traditional medical research method for studying individuals with problems is the *case study* method. More rigorous individual designs called *single-subject* experimental designs have been developed by behavioral psychologists for studying the effects of experimental treatments or training. The activities of individuals in natural settings may be studied by qualitative methods developed by anthropologists, sociologists, and phenomenological psychologists.

Recent interest in the pragmatic level of communication has required researchers to design studies of the communicative interactions of two or more persons. These designs may involve both qualitative and quantitative descriptions of verbal and nonverbal behaviors.

Description of Research Designs in Published Reports

Research designs are often described briefly at the end of the introductory section of published research reports, with further details of the design given in the second section, the *Method*. The description of the design may also be given in a subsection called *Design*, but is more often combined with the description of the procedure. The design must provide an acceptable means of achieving the stated purpose.

Examples of designs can be found in the first six reports in the June 1987 issue of JSHR. They are summarized here:

1. Detailed measures of sound masking were obtained for three subjects with HCDs and three non-HCD subjects with simulated HCDs under carefully controlled conditions.

2. Three tests of speech recognition were given to a group of 20 subjects with HCD on two occasions before and two occasions after a month of intensive auditory training.

3. Detailed measures of ear drum sound transmission were obtained for 127 adults without HCDs under carefully controlled conditions.

4. Two pairs of children with different kinds of articulation disorders were compared with each other and with children and adults without HCDs on detailed measures of tongue movement under carefully controlled conditions.

5. Twenty children with language disorders were compared with 20 children without HCDs on eight measures of communicative ability.

6. Nine adults with voice disorders were compared with 15 adults without HCDs on a large number of measures of vocal control.

These studies illustrate the types of designs used to achieve the purposes of HCD research.

THE PROCEDURE

The research design is an abstract description of the study. To put the design into practice, two further stages of planning are necessary. Decisions must be made about the exact procedure necessary to fulfill the requirements of the design. Then the researchers must determine whether resources are available to carry out the procedure. If not, the procedure and perhaps the design must be modified to fit the available resources. If this cannot be done, the study may have to be abandoned. Procedures used in HCD research are briefly described here, with more details given in Chapter 9.

Deciding on the Procedure

When the design has been made, it is necessary to decide exactly which subjects will be studied, what characteristics will be assessed, and how the assessments will be carried out. This aspect of research is just as important as the problem, the purpose, and the design of the study. The subjects have to be representative of the disordered and normal populations being studied, the characteristics assessed have to provide valid and reliable information about the processes studied, and the assessments have to be obtained in a well-controlled manner that rules out the possible influence of extraneous factors.

Determining Available Resources

The decisions concerning the procedure can only be put into action if the required resources are available. These include subjects with HCDs and subjects without HCDs, equipment and materials, facilities for assessment or training, and research personnel. The research personnel must be able to operate the equipment, make measurements, administer testing and training procedures required by the research, and analyze the results.

When the required resources are not available, the procedure must be modified or an attempt must be made to obtain them. For the types of research that are published as useful contributions to knowledge about HCDs, the necessary resources are often obtained by means of research grants from government agencies or private foundations.

Description of the Procedure in Published Reports

The procedure is described in the *Method* section of published research reports. Enough details should be given that someone else could repeat the study. As stated previously, the description of the procedure is often combined with the description of the design.

The subjects are usually described in a subsection entitled *Subjects*. Equipment and materials are described in subsections with headings such as *Tasks*, *Apparatus*, *Tests*, *Measures*, and *Instrumentation*. The operations for obtaining the required information about subjects are described in subsections with headings such as *Procedure*, *Test Procedure*, or *Training Procedure*. Examples of how the procedure is described in relation to the design can be found in the first six papers in the June 1987 issue of JSHR:

1. A lengthy procedure involving elaborate equipment was needed to measure the effects of tinnitus masking in six subjects.

2. Three speech recognition tests were given under carefully controlled conditions to 20 subjects one month before training, at the beginning and the end of one month's intensive training, and one month after training.

3. A lengthy procedure involving elaborate equipment was used to obtain detailed ear drum response measurements for 127 subjects.

4. Preliminary experience was given to eight subjects in wearing a specialized device for measuring tongue movement, and then very detailed measurements of tongue movement were obtained during a carefully controlled speech task.

5. Each of 40 subjects viewed a 45-minute filmed story and then told the story to two listeners and answered 30 questions about it.

6. Laryngeal movement in 24 subjects was measured by a special device during a carefully-controlled speech task.

These studies illustrate the procedures used in HCD research.

THE ANALYSIS

Data analysis is another essential research event. Even when resources are available for collecting the data, the researchers have to find appropriate methods for analyzing it, and must have the resources for carrying out the analysis, which can be very complex and time consuming. Where there are difficulties, fewer subjects may be studied or fewer measures obtained per subject. Data analyses are greatly facilitated by computer programs.

Where standard research designs are used, decisions about data analysis should be made at the same time as decisions about the design. The design may have to be changed if appropriate techniques of analysis are not available. Several different types of data analysis are possible. The type of analysis most appropriate for a particular study will depend on the purpose, the design, and the available procedures.

Before the information obtained in a study can be analyzed, it may be necessary to put the data into a different form. This stage of data analysis is called *data reduction*. Where data have been obtained by the judgments of observers, a preliminary analysis may be necessary to assess the reliability of the judgments. Then the analysis itself may involve numerical descriptions, statements of probability derived from statistical tests, or written descriptions. The different stages of analysis are briefly described here to indicate their place in the sequence of research events and will be described in more detail in Chapters 10 to 15.

Data Reduction

After the desired information has been collected in the manner prescribed by the procedure, it must be expressed in a way that is interpretable as evidence regarding the problem. Sometimes the information can be used in its original form; for example, the effects of a drug that causes hearing loss might be demonstrated by showing audiograms of several patients before and after administration of the drug. In most studies, however, one or more stages of data reduction are required.

Where information about communication has been recorded on audiotapes or videotapes, the data have to be transcribed into written form. This is a very time-consuming process, and resources may be available only for transcription of a restricted sample of the information. Judgments that put the transcribed responses into categories may be necessary for further analysis. This usually requires experienced judges and may be a lengthy process. It is often necessary to demonstrate reliability by statistical procedures that compare the transcriptions or judgments of two or more persons.

Where information is collected in the form of written narratives, categorical judgments and reliability estimates may also be necessary. Brief written or spoken responses can usually be categorized by the use of scoring rules. After responses have been placed in categories, they can be put into numerical form by counting the frequency of responses in each category. In qualitative analyses, different procedures would be used for further data analyses.

Numerical information derived from categorical judgments or from direct numerical measurements such as hearing thresholds can be further reduced by combining the detailed information into totals or averages that will be used for further analysis.

Descriptive Statistics

Numerical data can be presented in tables and graphs that give detailed information for individuals and groups. Interpretations can be directly based on this descriptive information. Descriptive statistics are used in almost all research reports, often as a supplement to inferential statistics. The detailed information provided by descriptive statistics can often be directly related to the concerns of practitioners.

Inferential Statistics

The numerical information in descriptive statistics can be further analyzed by inferential statistics to arrive at estimates of the probability that the observed effects would be found in other subjects of the same type. Statistical tests are used in group studies to assess differences between two or more groups, to assess change in one or more groups, and to determine the degree of relationship between the characteristics of a group.

Statistical tests require mathematical calculations of varying degrees of complexity. At one time, the lengthy calculations required by complex statistics made it impossible to carry out many studies, but computers have made even the most lengthy and complex analyses available to most researchers.

Qualitative Analyses

Analyses that do not require the transformation of data into numerical form may be appropriate for HCD research. Such analyses are directly based on written transcriptions of communicative interactions, interviews, or narratives. The methods of analysis include ethnographic methods taken from anthropology and interpretive methods taken from literary studies. They are called qualitative methods to distinguish them from quantitative analyses of numerical data.

The data of qualitative analyses are usually gathered in natural settings, and the research designs differ from those used in quantitative analyses. Qualitative analyses are becoming more common in HCD research with increased interest in the factors that influence communication in natural settings.

Description of Data Analyses in Published Reports

In published research reports, the techniques used for data analysis are often described in the *Method* section, sometimes in subsections entitled *Data Analysis*. The results of the data analysis are presented in the *Results* section. Descriptive and inferential statistics are usually presented in tables and graphs. Qualitative analyses are presented in written form.

Examples of quantitative analyses can be found in the first six papers of the June 1987 issue of JSHR. Numerical information was directly obtained in studies 1, 3, and 6; some test scoring was required in studies 2 and 4; and extensive transcription and interpretation were required in study 5. All six studies used descriptive statistics, and studies 2, 5, and 6 also used inferential statistics.

THE INTERPRETATION

After the data collected by researchers have been analyzed, the information provided by the analysis is evaluated in relation to the purpose of the study. Then the findings are related to the original problem, and conclusions are reached about the new information contributed by the research. Only rarely does the new information completely close the gap in practical knowledge that suggested the problem.

The interpretation can serve several very important functions. Conclusions may be reached regarding the extent to which the findings apply to others with HCDs, the implications of the findings for direct practical applications may be stated, and suggestions can be made for further research. More details regarding interpretation are given in Chapter 16.

In published research reports the interpretation is given in sections called *Discussion*, *Results and Discussion*, or *Discussion and Conclusions*. There are usually detailed descriptions of how the results relate to the problem and to previous research. The conclusions usually state the contribution of the findings to theoretical and practical knowledge, and are sometimes given in a separate section entitled *Conclusions* or *Implications*.

Examples of different types of discussion can be seen in the first six papers of the June 1987 issue of JSHR. The first three studies present conclusions concerning direct clinical applications of their findings, whereas the conclusions reached in the last three studies suggest that further research will lead to practical applications.

RESEARCH STRATEGIES

HCD research is seldom carried out under ideal circumstances. Previous research and theory rarely provide an exact definition of the gap in knowledge. Available research designs and methods of data analysis cannot always provide information directly applicable to HCDs. Subjects, materials, and facilities may not be available to meet the requirements of the research design and data analyses. Such limitations prevent researchers from obtaining all the information they need in one study. The findings may only suggest the kind of further research that should be done.

Under these circumstances, HCD researchers cannot simply be well-trained methodologists who apply a fixed set of techniques to achieve certain knowledge. They must be strategists who go as far as they can toward achieving their practical goals by whatever means are available. Many skills are needed for effective HCD research. Creativity is needed to identify an important problem, scholarship to search out previous theories and research, technical knowledge to make the plan and analyze the data, resourcefulness and diligent attention to detail to carry out the procedure, and interpretive abilities to explain the contribution to knowledge.

In addition to these separate skills, researchers must integrate the research events. The purpose has to fit the problem and the design; the design has to fit the purpose, the procedure, and the data analysis; the procedure has to fit the design and the available resources; and the data analysis has to fit the design, procedure, and purpose. To accomplish this integration, researchers have to be well informed, adaptable, ingenious, and highly goal oriented.

Although the chronicle of skills needed for HCD research is very lengthy, it is not greatly different from the set of skills needed for practice. Like professional practice, research requires knowledge, skill, and determination.

Description of Research Strategies in Published Reports

The published studies of successful HCD researchers show how research strategies are employed to achieve the practical goals of HCD research. The first six reports in the June 1987 issue of JSHR provide examples of research strategies employed for different types of problems:

1. Because the masking of tinnitus could be precisely measured, interpretations could be based on graphical results for the six subjects.

2. Because the effects of auditory training were relatively small and variable, statistical analysis of group data and careful interpretation were needed to conclude that the training resulted in practical benefits.

3. Ear drum responses of 127 normal subjects could be precisely measured to obtain tabular and graphic information that described the normal range of ear drum responses.

4. Tongue movements of four children with HCDs could be exactly compared on an individual basis with normal tongue movements, providing descriptive information concerning abnormal movements, inappropriate movements, and incorrectly sequenced movements.

5. Descriptions of a film by 20 non-HCD children and 20 language disordered children had to be transcribed, analyzed into linguistic categories, and statistically analyzed to reach conclusions concerning the effects of developmental language disorders on narrative discourse.

6. Detailed measures of the vocal movement control of nine patients with spasmodic dysphonia and nine subjects without spasmodic dysphonia were compared by statistical analyses to permit interpretation of the pattern of abnormal movement associated with spasmodic dysphonia.

These examples illustrate the research strategies required for different types of problems. No single strategy will suit all the different problems of HCD research.

The best way to become familiar with the kinds of strategies used in HCD research is to look at examples of research, as done in this chapter. A review of the brief descriptions of the problems, purposes, designs, procedures, data analyses, interpretations, and strategies used in the six studies will indicate how the events are integrated.

To understand how strategies are formulated, it is necessary to be familiar with the methods, procedures, and data analysis techniques of HCD research. A more detailed discussion of research strategies is given in Chapter 17, following the chapters on research designs, procedures, data analysis, and interpretation.

ADDITIONAL INFORMATION

Additional information regarding the sequence of research events is given in the books on HCD research listed at the end of Chapter 1, and in most introductory texts on psychological research (cf. Calfee, 1985).

REVIEW QUESTIONS

1. List the sequence of events in research, briefly describe each event, and indicate where they are described in research reports.
2. Find the research events in all of the research reports in a recent issue of the *Journal of Speech and Hearing Research* or the *Journal of Speech and Hearing Disorders*.

CHAPTER
3

Aspects of Human Communication Disorders Studied by Researchers

To understand the different events in HCD research, it is necessary to be familiar with the wide variety of problems studied by researchers. This chapter begins with a description of HCDs at each stage of communication. A series of 100 studies published in two leading journals will be surveyed to illustrate the aspects of HCDs that are investigated.

Communication is an ongoing exchange of information between two or more persons. It involves listening, understanding, formulating speech, and speaking. During communication, all of these activities are occurring at the same time. For descriptive purposes, however, it is convenient to consider them as successive stages. HCDs involve interference at one or more stages of communication.

LISTENING

Listening begins with the detection of sounds. Speech sounds must be discriminated from nonspeech sounds in order that the acoustic structure of speech can be integrated. Then the linguistic features, phonemes, words, and grammatical structure of speech can be perceived.

Detection

Sound vibrations are conducted through the ear drum and middle ear to the inner ear. Disorders at this stage are classified as *conductive hearing loss*. These disorders can occur as a result of heredity, disease, injury, or aging. The organic and behavioral changes are well understood.

Discrimination

Vibrations are transformed to nerve impulses in the inner ear. Acquired inner ear disorders are called *sensorineural hearing loss*, and congenital inner ear disorders are called *sensorineural hearing impairment*. These disorders can occur as a result of heredity, disease, injury, noise exposure, or aging. The organic and behavioral changes are relatively well understood.

Integration

Auditory nerve impulses are transmitted through a series of interconnected nerve cells in the midbrain to the auditory cortex of the temporal lobe. Disorders at this stage are called *central auditory disorders*. These disorders can occur as a result of disease or injury, and probably also as a result of heredity and sensory deprivation. The organic and behavioral changes are not well understood.

Perception

The integrated representation of speech is associated with stored "knowledge cues" (Elman & McLelland, 1984) to perceive linguistic features, phonemes, words, and grammatical structure. Disorders at this stage and the next two stages are usually considered *language disorders*, although it is not yet clear whether feature and phoneme disorders should be considered central auditory disorders. Language disorders may be acquired as a result of disease, injury, or aging, and probably also as a result of heredity, sensory deprivation, or inadequate experience. Language disorders acquired through brain dysfunction are called *aphasia*. Although there are interesting theories, disorders at the perceptual stage are not yet well understood.

Other Sensory Information

Visual information from lip movements, facial expressions, gestures, body postures, and signs may contribute to communication. Information from sound vibrations may be transmitted through the sense of touch. Researchers study the use of these other sensory inputs to help overcome listening problems, but visual and tactile disorders are not usually considered HCDs.

UNDERSTANDING

As words and syntactic structure are perceived, meaning is understood. Understanding can occur at the level of separate utterances, connected discourse, and communicative intentions (pragmatics). Developmental and acquired language disorders may involve any or all of these levels of understanding. There are interesting theories, but incomplete knowledge of language disorders.

FORMULATING SPEECH

The participants in communication listen, understand, and then formulate their own spoken contributions. Speech is formulated to express communicative intentions through connected discourse that is made up of individual utterances. Developmental and acquired language disorders may involve any or all levels of formulation. There are interesting theories, but incomplete knowledge of these disorders.

Theorists do not yet agree as to how language disorders involving perception, understanding, or formulating speech are related to type and location of brain dysfunction.

SPEAKING

As speech is formulated, it is spoken. Movements of the speech musculature, including the vocal cords, are planned and executed, resulting in speech sounds. A number of HCDs interfere with speech, including *dysarthria*, *dyspraxia*, *stuttering*, *voice disorders*, and *articulation/ phonological disorders*. The motor disorders of cerebral palsy also impair speech, as do the structural defects of cleft palate. Vocal cord function is impaired by surgery in laryngectomies. Speech disorders can occur as a result of heredity, disease, or injury. Some may also be the result of experiential factors. The disorders are usually easy to identify, but the exact patterns of impaired planning and execution of movements have not yet been completely described for most speech disorders.

Other Movements

Communicative expression also occurs through gestures, body movements, and signs. HCD researchers have studied these forms of expression as alternatives to speaking, but disorders of nonspeech movements are not usually considered HCDs.

SCOPE OF HCD RESEARCH

For certain disorders, there has been considerable research over the years. These disorders include stuttering, articulation disorders, voice disorders, cleft palate, aphasia, conductive hearing loss, sensorineural hearing loss, and congenital sensorineural hearing impairment. Research on both developmental and acquired language disorders has greatly increased in recent years, with the emphasis shifting from syntax to semantics to pragmatics as language theories have evolved. Research on central auditory disorders is still at a relatively early stage.

Researchers may concentrate on how a disorder directly affects communication, or on the indirect effects of disorders. For disorders such as stuttering, much of the research is concerned with its direct consequences for communication. For disorders such as early conductive hearing loss and congenital sensorineural hearing impairment, research may focus on how the disorders affect the development of communicative skills. Researchers may also be concerned with the effects of HCDs on factors such as personality and school achievement, and on the benefits of treatment or training.

Recent trends in HCD research demonstrate its scope and diversity, and provide a useful context for discussions of research events in later chapters. The following survey is based on 100 research reports published in 1986 and 1987 in the two leading North American HCD research journals. Consecutive reports were taken from the last three issues of 1986 and the first three issues of 1987 for the *Journal of Speech and Hearing Disorders* (JSHD), and from the last two issues of 1986 and the first two issues of 1987 of the *Journal of Speech and Hearing Research* (JSHR). The reports are listed according to the aspect of communication studied.

The published studies were almost equally divided between hearing (34 studies), language (35 studies), and speech (31 studies). Almost half were concerned with two disorders—acquired sensorineural disorders (22 studies) and developmental language disorders (24 studies). There were a number of studies of normal communication. Somewhat different trends would be revealed if research were surveyed over a different period and other journals were included.

HEARING

Almost all of the research on hearing was concerned with peripheral hearing disorders, either conductive or sensorineural.

Conductive Disorders (5 Studies)

There were studies of the normal range of tympanic membrane (ear drum) vibration (1), the tympanogram as an indicator of middle ear disease (2), the function of the acoustic reflex in the middle ear (1), and the possible effects on language development of conductive hearing loss in children (1).

Research on conductive disorders is also reported in audiology journals such as *Audiology*, *Ear and Hearing*, and the *Journal of Auditory Research*, as well as otolaryngology journals such as *Annals of Otology* and *Laryngoscope*.

Sensorineural Disorders (28 Studies)

Most of the research on hearing was concerned with acquired sensorineural hearing loss. There were studies of hearing measurement (3), hearing aid selection (5), self-evaluation of sensorineural loss (2), sensorineural loss in the aged (1), lipreading training (3), the transmission of pitch and loudness information (2), the transmission of phonetic information (1), the intelligibility of speakers who are hearing-impaired (1), training individuals with sensorineural hearing loss and blindness (1), and tinnitus (ringing in the ears) (3).

Research on acquired sensorineural hearing loss is also reported in audiology and otolaryngology journals.

Other research on sensorineural disorders concerned children with congenital sensorineural impairment. There were studies of hearing assessment (1), speech development (4), and language development (1).

Research on the assessment and training of children who are hearing-impaired is also reported in the *Volta Review* and the *American Annals of the Deaf*.

Central Auditory Disorders (1 Study)

The single study of central auditory disorders concerned behavioral measures for detecting tumors that affect the auditory nerve.

Research on central auditory disorders is also reported in audiology and otolaryngology journals.

LANGUAGE

Research on language is most usefully classified into acquired language disorders, developmental language disorders, and normal language, since many studies involve more than one stage of communication.

Acquired Language Disorders (5 Studies)

Research on aphasia included evaluation of language retraining of aphasics (1), studies of the effects of aphasia on discourse skills (3), and assessment of residual academic and language deficits in children with aphasia (1).

Research on acquired language disorders is also reported in *Brain and Language, Neuropsychologia*, and other neuropsychology and neurolinguistics journals.

Developmental Language Disorders (24 Studies)

Researchers studied the effects of developmental language disorders on auditory-visual abilities (1), awareness of speech sounds (1), learning new words (1), comprehension (1), discourse abilities (2), communicative intentions (pragmatic skills) (8), and cognitive strengths and weaknesses (1). There were studies that assessed a variety of treatment methods (8), and a study of the prevalence of developmental language disorders (1).

Research on developmental language disorders is also reported in a variety of linguistics, psycholinguistics, and neurolinguistics journals such as the *Journal of Applied Linguistics, Child Language*, and the *Journal of Communication Disorders.*

Normal Language (6 Studies)

Research on normal language included studies of speech-sound perception in normal listeners (1), the effects of aging on speech perception (1), the use of language in grouping objects (1), language used by mothers to their children (1), length of utterances by children (1), and communicative intentions of children (1).

Research on normal language is also reported in many linguistics, psycholinguistics, and neurolinguistics journals.

SPEECH

Research on speech disorders can be classified according to the type of disorder.

Voice Disorders (10 Studies)

There was research on laryngeal structures (2), laryngeal control (1), acoustic measurement (1), prediction of severity (1), clinicians' ability to judge voice disorders (1), methods for evaluating laryngectomees (3), and methods for improving speech in laryngectomees (1).

Other HCD research on voice disorders is reported in otolaryngology journals.

Articulation/Phonological Disorders (5 Studies)

Researchers studied articulation development (1), the effect of linguistic context on articulation (1), electrical measures of tongue movements (1), a test of articulation development (1), and a microcomputer test of articulation (1).

Other HCD research on articulation/phonological disorders is reported in the *Quarterly Journal of Speech* and the *Journal of Communication Disorders*.

Stuttering (7 Studies)

Research was concerned with word ending repetitions (1), prosodic disturbances (1), acoustic measures (1), electroglottal measures (1), right hemisphere mechanisms (1), linguistic complexity effects (1), and assertiveness training. (1)

HCD research on stuttering is also reported in the *Journal of Fluency Disorders*.

Cleft Palate (2 Studies)

Researchers studied a method of evaluating nasality (1) and a method of training articulation. (1)

Other HCD research on cleft palate is reported in the *Cleft Palate Journal*.

Dysarthria (1 Study)

Acoustic measures of dysarthria were reported in one study.

HCD research on dysarthria is also reported in otolaryngology, neurology, and physical medicine journals.

Normal Speech (6 Studies)

Research using normal subjects included studies of tongue movement (1), lip movement (1), reflex responses of jaw (1), lip (1), and tongue (1), interaction of speech and finger movements (1), relation of body type to speech breathing (1), and effects of noise and filtering on speech (1).

Research on normal speech is also published in the *Journal of Phonetics* and the *Journal of the Acoustical Society of America*.

ADDITIONAL INFORMATION

Additional information about aspects of HCDs studied by researchers is best obtained by looking through current issues of *JSHR*, *JSHD*, and other HCD journals.

REVIEW QUESTIONS

1. List the stages of human communication and the HCDs at each stage.
2. Take recent issues of *JSHR* and *JSHD*, and classify each research report according to the stage of communication and the type of HCD studied.
3. Classify research reports in recent issues of more specialized journals such as the *Journal of Fluency Disorders* and *Ear and Hearing* according to the stage of communication and the type of HCD studied.

CHAPTER

4

Basic Principles of Research Design

To select an important problem, researchers must know about human communication and be aware of gaps in knowledge. Then a study is designed to accomplish a specific purpose related to the problem. Special knowledge about designs applicable to HCD research is required. This technical knowledge is a basic tool of HCD research.

The problems of HCD research require a variety of research designs. The types of design available to HCD researchers are described in Chapters 5 to 8. Designs that achieve the purposes of HCD research have been borrowed from several disciplines. Standard psychological research designs permit statistical analysis of differences between and within groups of subjects. Some of these designs have been specially adapted for practical problems. Designs for studying individuals have been borrowed from several sources, including case history methods from medicine, single-subject designs from psychology, and qualitative methods from anthropology and sociology.

A single book cannot provide all of the technical details of the different designs used in HCD research. For each type of research design discussed in the following chapters, references are given to texts and articles that provide more detailed technical information. Even if complete information about all designs could be given, knowledge of design techniques is not enough. Researchers must know how to combine and adapt available designs to achieve the practical purposes of HCD research. Strategies used in the thoughtful planning of HCD research are described in Chapter 17.

Underlying the designs and strategies are certain basic principles of research design. These principles will be discussed in this chapter.

CONTROLS

Theorists increase our understanding of HCDs by creative integration of present knowledge. Researchers obtain new knowledge about HCDs by observation. Research designs are the rules for observation. The rules for observation of parent-child communication in natural settings are quite different from the rules for laboratory observation of very restricted aspects of ear drum or tongue movement. A detailed explanation of *controls* and *variables* is essential to an understanding of the basic principles or rules of research design.

A control is a restriction of natural variation. Research designs control natural variations to isolate the variables that are to be studied. The variables that are controlled in HCD research include characteristics of the *subjects* who participate in the research and characteristics of the *situation* in which the observations are made. Control of the subject and situational variables permits researchers to study the effects of the variables in which they are interested.

The extent to which each kind of variation is controlled depends on the research design. Since HCD research is designed to achieve practical goals, complete control of all variables except the variables of interest is seldom achieved. As a result, HCD researchers must be extremely cautious in interpreting their findings. An important aspect of interpretation is to evaluate the extent to which all relevant variables have been controlled.

Subject Controls

The type of HCD to be studied is controlled by the selection of subjects who have that type of HCD. To isolate the effects of the HCD, subjects of a certain age, sex, cultural background, education, and history of treatment may be studied. In such a case, these subject variables are controlled by holding them constant. If these variables were not controlled, attempts to study the effects of the HCD might be *confounded* by the effects of the uncontrolled variables.

Another control procedure is to compare subjects with HCDs to subjects without HCDs. The control subjects are commonly formed into groups called *control groups*. The control group is matched with a group of HCD subjects on variables such as age, sex, and cultural background. To the extent that the groups can be matched on *relevant variables*, the effects of the HCD will be isolated. To the extent that all relevant variables are not controlled, the effects of the HCD are not completely isolated.

All HCD research does not involve the comparison of HCD groups and control groups. Some designs compare only groups of HCD subjects differing in type of HCD, age, sex, history of treatment, or other variables. Relevant variables are also controlled in the selection of such groups. Other designs involve repeated measurements of a single group. The controls required for such designs will be discussed later. Still other designs study individuals rather than groups. In such designs, the interpretation of differences between individuals depends on the extent to which relevant variables have been controlled.

Situation Controls

In addition to subject variables, the research design controls the situation. If the variable studied is the detection of sounds, sounds will be presented under carefully controlled acoustic conditions where background noise and reverberation are kept to a minimum to isolate the effect of the experimental sound. If the variable studied is stuttering, the speech situation may be controlled by the use of a standardized interview to reduce the possibility that the amount and type of stuttering are influenced by situational variability.

Other variables such as time of day and instructions to subjects may also be controlled. The situational controls depend on the information about HCDs that is being sought. Where an observer is present who records observations, controls may be necessary to rule out the possibility that the observer's expectations will affect the observations. Likewise, it may be necessary to control the possibility that the observations will be affected by the subjects' expectations.

The need for situational controls varies with the type of design. Researchers who wish to determine how sounds are detected in real-life situations will not control background noise and reverberation. Similarly, researchers who wish to assess stuttering in natural situations will not restrict observations to carefully controlled speaking situations. Even in natural situations, however, some control is exerted. HCD researchers studying communication in natural settings would usually observe only situations in which communication is likely to occur, and perhaps exert some control over the situation. The caregiver may be asked to play with the child who is being observed, in order that a particularly important form of natural communication may be observed.

Controls are essential for achieving the purposes of research. If the variables under study are not isolated by controlling relevant variables, alternative explanations of the findings cannot be ruled out. For example, to determine whether children with language disorders are deficient in speech sound perception, it is necessary to rule out the possibilities that observed differences in speech perception are not a function of age, sex, linguistic background, hearing impairment, the acoustic and linguistic characteristics of the speech sounds, the listening conditions, and the expectancies of the subjects and observers.

Decisions regarding which variables to control are extremely important. Where necessary controls have not been applied, the purpose of research may not be accomplished. Many reports of unexpected causes and miraculous cures have raised false hopes, because observations were not based on a research design that controlled relevant variables.

VARIABLES

Control and variability represent the opposite extremes of order and disorder. Both are essential to research. In carefully controlled studies, subject and situation variables are controlled. Only the phenomena of interest are allowed to vary. The variables that have been described previously as "phenomena of interest," "experimental treatments," and "the variable under study" are those whose effects are isolated by controlling relevant variables. The technical term for these variables is *independent variable*. The technical term for the observed effects of varying the independent variables is *dependent variable*. To understand how research designs work, it is necessary to fully understand these terms.

Independent Variables

Research designs are rules about controls and variables, and controlled variation. The terminology can be confusing. Researchers systematically vary the independent variable by controlling its variation. Research design is described in terms of the systematic variation of the independent variables, the observation of the effects of the independent variables on the dependent variables, and the systematic control of other variables that might produce variation in the dependent variables. The researcher varies independent variables to observe their effects on dependent variables.

Through all of these descriptions runs the idea that independent variables provide the information that fill gaps in knowledge about HCDs.

The aspect of the independent variable that is varied by the research design is the *level* of the independent variable. The levels can involve quantitative or qualitative variations. Quantitative variations could be different age levels or different levels of background masking noise. Qualitative variations could be subjects of different sexes or different types of communication situation. The effects of two or more levels of an independent variable and of two or more independent variables can be studied. In this way, complex, multidimensional information about HCDs can be obtained by a single experimental design.

Like control variables, independent variables can be subject variables or situation variables. Examples of independent subject variables are HCD versus non-HCD, treatment (or training) versus no treatment, type of treatment, type of HCD, age, sex, cultural background, and history of treatment. Examples of independent situation variables are before versus after treatment, different levels of language ability, sound frequency, masking noise, and different communication situations. All such variables can either be held constant as controlled variables or systematically varied as independent variables, depending on the purpose of the research.

Even in naturalistic observation, independent variables can be identified. In research where the purpose is to learn about the everyday communication of children who stutter, the independent variables could include comparison of stutterers of different ages and sexes, and comparison of different communication situations.

Dependent Variables

The outcome of the controls and variations exerted by research designs is variation in the dependent variables. Variations in dependent variables are recorded by quantitative or qualitative observations. In studies of voice disorders, the dependent variables might be quantitative acoustic measures or qualitative perceptual judgments of hoarseness or breathiness. In research on hearing, the dependent variables might be quantitative measures of hearing thresholds at different frequencies or qualitative judgments by hearing impaired subjects of their feelings about being hearing impaired. In research on language disorders, the dependent variables might be quantitative judgments of the syntactic complexity of written stories or qualitative descriptions of communicative interactions.

Both quantitative and qualitative dependent variables can be observed in the same study. In analyzing communicative interactions, both the frequency of each type of interchange and the patterns or themes that emerge can be recorded. Different types of dependent variable can also be observed in the same study. In comparisons between children without disorders and children with articulation/phonological disorders, not only speech but tongue, lip, and jaw movements can be observed.

The data provided by dependent variables are evaluated and interpreted to determine how much knowledge about HCDs has been obtained. The amount of confidence that can be placed in the findings depends in part on how well the design has controlled relevant variables and isolated the effects of independent variables. It also depends on the extent to which the design is appropriate to the problem, and on the repeatability of the observations. The design is evaluated in terms of *validity* and the observations are evaluated in terms of *reliability*. These are the two remaining principles of research design to be considered in this chapter.

VALIDITY AND RELIABILITY

The independent and dependent variables in an experimental design are carefully selected to achieve new knowledge. The knowledge will be most helpful if the measure of the dependent variable is both reliable and valid. A measure is *valid* to the extent that it measures what it claims to measure, and *reliable* to the extent that it is consistent and repeatable.

Validity

The two kinds of validity that are most important for HCD research are *internal validity* and *external validity*. A study is internally valid when relevant variables have been controlled, and the only variables that affect the dependent variables are the independent variables. When uncontrolled variables can affect the dependent variable, the effects of the independent variable are *confounded* with the effects of the uncontrolled variables. For example, if the effects of age and other relevant variables are not controlled, a study of the effects of lipreading training on communicative competence may be confounded. The success of standard research designs depends on the control of variables that might confound the effects of the independent variables.

External validity is the extent to which the effects of independent variables on dependent variables in the research situation apply to the natural setting. How does the ability of hearing impaired children to repeat isolated words relate to the intelligibility of their speech in natural settings? If the information obtained by research does not have external validity, it may not be of immediate practical use.

Reliability

Measurements of dependent variables are reliable to the extent that the same measurements would be obtained if the study were repeated. If the measures are numerical scores, it may be important to estimate how much the scores would vary if the test were repeated. If the measurements are judgments by an observer, it may be necessary to determine whether other observers would make the same judgments. Any source of inconsistency that produces variation in the measurement of the independent variables may confound the effects of the independent variables. The reliability of measurements can be estimated in several ways. *Test-retest reliability* is assessed by obtaining the same measurement twice and comparing the two measurements. *Split-half reliability* can be assessed when measurements consist of a series of items. The items are split in half and the resulting measurements compared. *Alternate form reliability* can be assessed when alternative forms of measurement are compared. *Observer reliability* is assessed when the judgments of two or more observers are compared.

Both reliability and validity must be taken into consideration in designing and interpreting experiments that are intended to provide useful information about HCDs.

BASIC PRINCIPLES OF HCD RESEARCH

One of the most crucial aspects of HCD research is the thoughtful selection of the variables that are to be controlled or systematically varied. After a problem has been found and the purpose specified, there must be careful consideration of which variables are most relevant to the problem and the purpose. HCDs are complex, and the relevant variables for research on HCDs are not always obvious. Where relevant variables are not taken into consideration, many years of research can be wasted, and practical applications of the research findings may have unfortunate consequences for persons with HCDs.

Most HCD research designs do not just involve one independent variable, one dependent variable, and a small set of controlled variables. Rather than hold age and sex constant in studying the language skills of children who are hearing impaired, the researcher may wish to determine the effects of age and sex on language skill by systematically varying them. Likewise, the researcher may not obtain sufficient information to achieve the purpose of assessing the language skills of children who are hearing impaired by observing one type of language skill, but may wish to observe the effects of hearing impairment on vocabulary, grammar, and connected discourse.

The purpose of the research governs the selection of the independent and dependent variables. The research design prescribes reliable observations that will lead to valid conclusions concerning the effects of the independent variables on the dependent variables. A clear understanding of the functions of controls and variables and the concepts of reliability and validity is the key to understanding the basic principles of research design. These principles apply to all types of research.

The amount and type of control and variation and the need to demonstrate reliability and validity depend on the aspects of HCDs studied and the purpose of the research. Researchers must familiarize themselves with the different kinds of research designs in order to select those most appropriate for the problems they wish to study. The function of controls and variables in research designs is most easily illustrated in the simple group research designs borrowed from psychological research, as described in the next chapter.

ADDITIONAL INFORMATION

Basic principles of research design can be found in recent texts by Ray and Ravizza (1985) and Calfee (1985). Standard terminology has been defined in a comprehensive reference book by Yaremko, Harari, Harrison, and Lynn (1986). More complete discussions of validity and reliability can be found in texts dealing with psychological testing (cf. Anastasi, 1982).

REVIEW QUESTION

Briefly define the following terms: *controls, variables, subject controls, situation controls, confounding, relevant variables, independent variables, levels of independent variables, dependent variables, validity, reliability, internal validity, external validity, test-retest reliability, split-half reliability, alternate form reliability, observer reliability.*

EXERCISES (answers are given in Appendix D)

1. Researchers wish to find out if children with speech production disorders also have difficulty understanding speech. They give a speech perception test to a group of children with articulation disorders and a group of children without articulation disorders. The test consists of 50 items, each of which requires the child to point to one of three pictures that represent a spoken word.

a. List relevant subject and situation controls.
b. Give an example of confounding the effects of articulation disorders by an uncontrolled variable.
c. What are the independent and the dependent variables?
d. What are the levels of the independent variable?
e. How would internal validity and external validity be determined?
f. How could the reliability of the speech perception test be determined?
g. Would it be necessary to assess observer reliability? (explain)

2. Researchers wish to evaluate a new treatment for stuttering. They record a speech sample from a group of stutterers before and after training.

a. What are the independent and dependent variables?
b. What are the levels of the independent variable?
c. How would external validity be determined?
d. Should reliability be assessed ? (If so, say what type and how)

3. Researchers wish to evaluate a new treatment of stuttering. They record speech samples from a group of stutterers who have been given a new type of training and a group of stutterers who have not been given the new type of training.

a. What are the independent and dependent variables?
b. What are the levels of the independent variable?
c. List relevant subject and situation controls.
d. Which group is the control group?
e. Give an example of confounding the effects of training by an uncontrolled variable.

CHAPTER
5

Simple Group Research Designs

G roup research designs isolate the effects of independent variables by controlling for the inherent variability of human behavior. Behavior is much more variable than physiological processes. The operation of the circulatory, respiratory, and digestive systems is more uniform in all persons. Physiologists record responses that do not vary greatly from one person to another under standard laboratory conditions. As a result, they can obtain knowledge of human physiology by carefully controlled observations of a small number of individuals.

Human behavior varies greatly as a function of a host of variables, including age, sex, personality, education, culture, and individual life experience. Even under the most standard laboratory conditions, there will be individual differences in the behaviors studied. Researchers attempt to overcome this variability by estimating the probability that one set of carefully controlled observations is different from another set of carefully controlled observations.

Research concerned with the physiological aspects of HCDs does not usually require standard group research designs. A great deal of HCD research does, however, involve the kind of variable behavior for which group designs were developed. Even then, group designs may not be appropriate. Information about groups is not always suitable to the practical purposes of HCD research.

Simple group designs are described in this chapter, complex group designs are described in Chapter 6, and the advantages and disadvantages of group research designs for HCD research are discussed in Chapter 7. The simplest group designs involve one independent variable with two levels, and one dependent variable. The levels of the independent variable can be independent groups or repeated measurements. These two types of design will be discussed separately.

INDEPENDENT GROUP DESIGNS

In simple independent group designs the independent variable has two levels, represented by two independent groups. There are four types of independent group designs—random selection, random assignment, matched group, and natural group designs. The natural group design is most commonly used in HCD research.

Random Selection Designs

The most basic design is the random selection design for two groups. The groups are randomly selected from the same population. There is one independent variable with two levels, and one dependent variable. One group receives one level of the independent variable and the other group receives the other level. The effect of varying the independent variable is indicated by the difference between groups on the dependent variable.

Variables such as age, sex, and education are controlled by random selection of subjects, which ensures that there will be no systematic differences between groups for these variables. Situation variables are held as constant as possible for all subjects in both groups. When these simple rules of research design have been followed, a statistical analysis can be carried out to estimate the probability that the value of the dependent variable for Group 1 differs from that for Group 2, thus accomplishing the purpose of the research.

For example, two groups of 100 children are randomly selected from the total population of children with language disorders. The independent variable is vocabulary training. One group is given extensive training in which new words are introduced in the context of stories and the other group is given no training. Then both groups take a vocabulary test that includes the new words. The score on the vocabulary test is the dependent variable. Subject variables such as age, sex, and education are controlled by allowing them to vary randomly. Situation variables such as testing room, time of testing, and the person giving the vocabulary test are held constant. The difference between groups in vocabulary test scores is evaluated by statistical analysis to estimate the effect of training in defining words on the vocabularies of children with language disorders.

This standard design is described by standard terms. The *independent variable* is the *treatment*. The two *levels* of the treatment are vocabulary training and no vocabulary training. The group receiving the treatment is the *experimental group* and the group receiving no treatment is the *control group*. The term *control* is also applied to situational variables that are held constant for both groups. The measure of the effect of the treatment (vocabulary test score) is the *dependent variable*.

A group research design was used to study the effects of vocabulary training. Vocabulary is a variable psychological process. With the simple random group design, the independent variable was isolated by a random selection procedure that controlled subject variables. Careful control of the experimental situation ensured that relevant variables other than the independent variable were held constant. Then the effect of the independent variable could be demonstrated by differences between groups on the dependent variable.

If the rules of this simple design are followed, the researcher can evaluate the effects of training in a rigorous, scientifically acceptable manner. Such a design could be very useful for HCD researchers. However, random selection from an entire population of either HCD or non-HCD populations is virtually impossible for HCD researchers. Even if it were not, many researchers would prefer to systematically control variables such as age, sex, and education rather than allowing them to vary randomly.

Random Assignment Designs

Random assignment designs overcome the difficulty of access to an entire population. When only a restricted population of subjects is available, they can be randomly assigned to one group or the other. Like the random selection procedure, subject variables are controlled by allowing them to vary randomly. Except for the population from which subjects are selected, there is no difference between random selection and random assignment designs. All of the other characteristics of random selection designs apply to random assignment designs.

Random assignment designs are more feasible than random selection designs for HCD research. The researcher can randomly assign two groups from whatever population is available. However, the design has potential drawbacks. The restricted population from which the subjects are selected may not be representative of the entire population. For example, a group of children with language disorders from one city may differ in cultural and linguistic background from the entire population of children with language disorders. In such a case, the research findings would only apply to language disorders with the characteristics of that particular population.

Another potential difficulty with random assignment designs is that the relatively small populations available for random selection may be extremely variable. Subjects may differ greatly in relevant subject variables. In such cases, the dependent variable might vary a great deal as a function of these subject variables. The variability within groups and between groups might obscure the effect of the independent variable. For example, randomly assigned groups of children with language disorders might vary greatly in vocabulary as a function of age, education, cultural background, and language background. Such variation might be quite large relative to the variation resulting from the vocabulary training of one group.

Matched Group Designs

The subject variability that may be a problem in random assignment designs can be overcome by matched group designs. In the simple matched group design one or more variables that may affect the dependent variable can be held constant between groups by matching the groups on those variables. There are two types of matched group design. In treatment studies, the two groups can be matched on the dependent variable prior to treatment. They are selected in such a way that both groups have the same average score on the dependent variable. For example, in a vocabulary training study the two groups can be matched on the basis of a vocabulary test given prior to training. Then, any differences between groups in vocabulary after training can be attributed to the independent variable, training versus nontraining.

In the other type of matched group design, groups are matched on variables other than the dependent variable. Variables are selected for matching that might affect the dependent variable, such as age, sex, and education. This matching procedure, like the pretreatment matching procedure described previously, should help to isolate the effects of the independent variable. Differences between groups matched on relevant variables should reflect the effects of the independent variable. If two groups could not be matched in vocabulary prior to training, they could be matched in age, sex, education, and cultural background to control the effects of these variables on the dependent variable. Then any differences between groups in vocabulary could be more clearly attributed to the independent variable of training.

The final consideration for matched group designs is the exact form of matching. If two groups are to be matched in vocabulary, the minimum requirement is that both groups have the same average vocabulary prior to training. Variability in pretraining vocabulary can be reduced even further if the distribution of vocabulary scores around the mean (group average) is the same for both groups. Then the more restricted the distribution, the better will be the control of pretraining vocabulary. The effects of vocabulary training are more easily demonstrated for groups whose pretraining vocabularies vary within a very limited range.

The same reasoning holds true for matching on other variables. Not only the average age but the distribution of ages of the two groups should be the same, and the best control of age is for both groups to be at a single age level. This is most important in studies of infants and young children, where there are large developmental changes. Both groups should have the same proportion of boys and girls, and sex effects are best controlled if all subjects are of the same sex. Similarly, education and cultural background are best controlled if all subjects are at the same education level and come from the same cultural background. These restrictions in the range of variation of matched variables will enhance the observed effects of the independent variable.

The matched group design is very appropriate for HCD research, because the relatively small populations available to most researchers make it very difficult to select comparable groups by random assignment. In matched group designs, like random selection and random assignment designs, the independent and dependent variables are clearly defined and other variables that may affect the dependent variable are controlled. What is sacrificed in the simple matched group design as compared with the random selection design is the ability to generalize the findings to the entire population. If all subjects are of the same age, sex, education, and cultural background, the findings may not apply to subjects of other ages, sexes, education levels, and cultural backgrounds. Designs that help to overcome problems of restricted generality are discussed in the next chapter.

Natural Group Designs

The remaining type of simple independent group design is the natural group design. In this design, the groups are selected from two different populations. The designs previously discussed select two groups from the same population, and the independent variable is different treatment of the two groups. In the natural group design, the independent variable is a difference between groups "created by nature" that exists prior to the selection of the groups. The effect of this independent variable is studied. Other variables that might affect the dependent variable are controlled by random selection or by matching.

For example, a randomly selected group of boys can be compared with a randomly selected group of girls in their performance on a vocabulary test to determine whether girls have better vocabularies than boys. The independent variable is sex, the dependent variable is once again vocabulary score, and all other variables are uncontrolled.

An important limitation of the natural group design is that the groups may differ in subtle ways that are not easy to detect or to control. Differences between groups may be attributable to these uncontrolled variables rather than to the independent variable. In the comparison of girls and boys, differences in vocabulary might be attributable to different cultural attitudes toward girls and boys rather than to natural (i.e., biological or organic) differences.

Combined Natural Group and Matched Group Designs

A design commonly used in HCD research is the combined matched group and natural group design. The restricted samples of HCD subjects available to researchers usually rule out random selection and assignment, making it necessary to match groups on relevant variables. In studies where HCD groups are compared with normal control groups, the natural group design must be used, because the two groups come from different populations. This is also true of comparisons between HCD groups that differ in type or severity of HCD, or in other variables such as age and sex. Because the combined matched group and natural group design is so important for HCD research, several examples will be given.

It may be important to determine whether children with observable articulation/phonological disorders also have higher-level language disorders. Higher-level language skills of a natural group of children with articulation disorders and a natural group of children without articulation disorders would be compared. The independent variable would be the presence of articulation disorders. The dependent variable would be a measure of higher-level language skill (e.g., a vocabulary test or a grammar test). A restricted group of children with articulation disorders would be available. The control group of children without articulation disorders would be selected to match the articulation disorder group in relevant variables such as age, sex, education, and cultural background.

If all relevant variables had been controlled, a difference between groups on the measure of higher-level language skill would provide evidence that children with articulation disorders do have higher-level language disorders. However, the difference might be attributable to variables other than articulation *per se*, such as organic or environmental factors associated with articulation disorders. It could not, therefore, be concluded that there is a cause-and-effect relationship between articulation disorders and higher-level language disorders. All that can be concluded is that children with articulation disorders tend to have higher-level language disorders, for whatever reason.

There is another difficulty in drawing conclusions about the cause-and-effect relationship between higher-level language disorders and articulation disorders. In random selection designs that have the necessary situation controls, it can be concluded that the independent variable has caused a change in the dependent variable. The causes of HCDs cannot be determined by simple natural group designs. Even if all relevant variables had been controlled, there would be no way of proving that the articulation disorders had not been caused by the higher-level language disorder, or that both disorders had not been separately caused by another disorder such as dysfunction of the left cerebral hemisphere. Difficulties in reaching conclusions about cause-and-effect relationships are discussed further in Chapter 7.

Natural/matched group designs can also be used to compare two groups of HCDs where the natural groupings are defined by differences in experience. A study may be designed to assess the effects of different methods of training children with congenital sensorineural hearing impairment. A group trained by auditory oral methods and a group trained by total communication methods would be compared in educational achievement. The independent variable would be method of language training and the dependent variable a measure of educational achievement especially adapted for children who are hearing-impaired. Variables controlled by matching might include age, sex, years of education, cultural background, amount of hearing impairment, and time of beginning language training.

If all relevant variables could be controlled by matching, differences between groups in educational achievement might be attributed to the method of language training. However, even when the "natural" grouping variable is a difference in experience, it is difficult to control all possibly relevant variables. For example, the two training methods may not be equally available, and the selection of a training method may be influenced by variables such as the child's aptitudes and the attitudes of parents and professionals toward the training methods. Differences between natural groups might be the results of such variables rather than the training methods themselves.

The simple matched/natural groups design is often suitable for the purposes of HCD research, but its limitations must be clearly recognized. Matching groups restricts the applicability of the results to groups with the same characteristics, it is difficult to match natural groups on all relevant variables, and a difference between natural groups does not prove that the independent variable has caused the difference. These are very important restrictions for researchers who are trying to fill gaps in knowledge.

REPEATED MEASUREMENT DESIGNS

In the independent group designs described earlier, the independent variable is a difference in the treatment of two groups. In the second type of simple group design, the two levels of the independent variable are varied within a single group of subjects. These designs are called *repeated measurement* or *within-group* designs. They are used in HCD research when there are not enough subjects available for two independent groups, when it is difficult to match relevant variables in two independent groups, or when it is more efficient to carry out the experimental procedures with one group. Simple repeated measurement designs may be more appropriate than simple independent group designs for studying the effects of training and for studying changes over time in the dependent variable. The latter studies are called *longitudinal studies*.

The basic rules of the repeated measurement design are simple. The dependent variable is assessed twice in a single group of subjects. The difference between the two assessments demonstrates the effect of the independent variable. Subject variables such as age, sex, and education do not have to be controlled, because the same group is used for both values of the independent variable.

Two examples illustrate the usefulness of this design for HCD research. If the purpose is to compare the effectiveness of two types of hearing aid, pure tone thresholds can be measured in a group of adults who are hearing-impaired with each kind of hearing aid. The relative effectiveness of the hearing aids is determined by the difference in average aided hearing thresholds. The independent variable is hearing aids and the dependent variable is average aided threshold for each aid. There is no need to control subject variables, since the same subjects are tested with both aids, but the conditions of testing the two aids must be exactly the same.

The second example involves the evaluation of training. To determine the effects of vocabulary training on children who are language impaired, a single group of children can be given the vocabulary test before and after training. The difference between pretraining and posttraining vocabulary indicates the effectiveness of vocabulary training. The independent variable is vocabulary training and the dependent variable is vocabulary test score before and after training. There is no need to control subject variables, but the conditions for pre- and posttraining vocabulary tests should be exactly the same.

Repeated measurement designs have several advantages over independent group designs, but they have their own limitations. In both of the previous examples, the repeated measurement of the dependent variable may be affected by the original measurement, and thus confound the effect of the independent variable. Repeated measurement effects are called *order effects*. Order effects may take the form of a practice effect that improves performance or a fatigue or boredom effect that impairs performance. When repeated measurement designs are used to assess the effects of training, there is a lack of control for the possibility that improvement might have occurred without training, that is, the lack of the control group with no training.

To control for order effects in the first example, thresholds should be measured first with one hearing aid for half the subjects and first with the other hearing aid for the other half. This is a control procedure called *counterbalancing* the order of presentation. Counterbalancing cannot be used to control for order effects in training studies, because the pretraining test must always be the first measure.

Even though counterbalancing eliminates confounding by order effects, variability resulting from large order effects could obscure the effect of the independent variable. Such variability can be reduced by extensive practice before the final measurements are made.

To control for the possibility of improvement without training, the independent group and repeated measure design can be combined, with a trained and an untrained group tested before and after training. This complex design will be discussed in the next chapter.

NUMBER OF SUBJECTS NEEDED
FOR SIMPLE GROUP DESIGNS

It would be helpful if the number of subjects needed for a given design could be specified in advance. In general, the more subjects the better, provided their characteristics meet the requirements of the design. However, where it is difficult to find subjects with the desired characteristics, some guidelines regarding the minimum number of subjects are needed.

The minimum number of subjects for studying treatment effects depends on the expected size of the effect and the expected variability within groups, plus other factors that will be discussed in the chapters on data analysis. The smaller the expected treatment effect and the larger the expected within-group variance, the more subjects are needed.

At the time research is being designed, it is helpful to have some information about treatment effects and within-group variance to estimate whether it is feasible to carry out the study with available subjects. In the absence of such information, a very rough estimate of the minimum number of subjects for simple group designs is 20. This would require 10 subjects for each of the two groups in independent group designs and 20 subjects for the one group in repeated measurement designs.

A desirable minimum for simple group designs would be 20 subjects. In HCD research where subjects are extremely difficult to obtain, an absolute minimum for simple group designs would be 10 subjects. Such small numbers of subjects may be appropriate for *pilot studies* that are intended to provide preliminary information for use in planning further research. Studies with small groups of subjects are not usually accepted for publication in research journals. An alternative to small groups would be the use of designs that do not require groups, as discussed in Chapter 8.

SIMPLE CORRELATION DESIGNS

Another common group design is the correlation design. In its simplest form, two different measures are obtained from each subject in a single group for the purpose of determining the relationship between the measures. For example, it may be important to determine the relationship between language ability and reading achievement in children who are hearing impaired. A measure of language ability and a measure of reading achievement are obtained for a group of children who are hearing impaired. A statistical analysis indicates the degree of relationship or *correlation* between the two measures. This provides an estimate of the extent to which good reading is associated with good language ability and poor reading with poor language ability.

Books on research design may not discuss correlation designs as such. Correlations are less definite than differences between experimental conditions. The independent and dependent variables are not usually defined. The degree of relationship estimates the similarity of two variables rather than the difference between two levels of an independent variable.

A major limitation of correlation designs is the difficulty in interpreting the observed relationships. In the previous example, the researchers might wish to find out whether reading difficulties of children who are hearing-impaired are caused by their difficulties in language acquisition. However, a high correlation between language ability and reading achievement is not sufficient evidence of a cause-and-effect relationship. It is conceivable that reading difficulties cause language difficulties, or that both variables are correlated with a third variable such as age. The degree of relationship also depends on the amount of variability among subjects for the two measures. Where there is restricted variability the correlation may be smaller.

Because of these limitations, correlation designs are often used to provide supplementary evidence rather than primary evidence regarding a particular HCD research problem.

ADDITIONAL INFORMATION

Simple research designs are discussed in texts on research methods in psychology. Shaughnessy and Zechmeister (1985) have given a very clear explanation of simple group designs. Other recent texts on research methods, in addition to those listed in Chapter 4, include Elmes, Kantowitz, and Roediger (1984), Martin (1985), and Sommer and Sommer (1986). Solso and Johnson (1984) have employed a case approach which makes use of examples of published studies.

REVIEW QUESTIONS

1. List the simple group designs discussed in this chapter.
2. Briefly define each design.
3. Give the main limitations of each type of research design for HCD research.

EXERCISES (answers are given in Appendix D)

1. In simple group designs, how many independent variables, levels of independent variables, and dependent variables are there?

2. What is the minimum number of subjects for simple independent group designs?

3. What kind of designs were used in Exercises 1, 2, and 3 in Chapter 4?

4. What would be the most appropriate type of simple group design for the following problems:

Possible personality problems of stutterers

Evaluation of a new speech aid for laryngectomees

Comparison of two speech discrimination tests

5. You wish to determine whether a new hearing aid is better than a standard hearing aid for children who are hearing-impaired. Identify the independent variable, the levels of the independent variable, the dependent variable, and relevant subject and situation controls. Design studies of this problem using random assignment, matched group, and repeated measurement designs.

CHAPTER

6

Complex Group Research Designs

In simple group designs there is one independent variable with two levels, and one dependent variable. Such designs can yield useful information about HCDs, as described in the previous chapter. However, the information may be limited. Complex designs can provide more detailed information about HCDs. The complex designs described in this chapter are based on the simple designs described in the previous chapter.

Complex designs are logical extensions of simple designs. There may be more than two levels of the independent variable, and more than one independent variable. There may also be more than one dependent variable. Independent group designs and repeated measure designs may be combined. All of this results in a large number of possible designs to serve the variety of purposes of HCD research. Complex group designs make many more research tools available to HCD researchers.

DESIGNS WITH MORE THAN TWO LEVELS
OF THE INDEPENDENT VARIABLE

In simple group designs the independent variable has two levels. The two levels used in the examples in the previous chapter were vocabulary training versus no training, boys versus girls, articulation/phonological disorders versus normal speech, auditory oral versus total communication methods, hearing aid 1 versus hearing aid 2, and pretraining versus post-training vocabulary. Researchers often wish to assess more than two levels of the independent variable. For example, more information about age effects is obtained by assessing three or more age levels in independent group designs, and more complete information is obtained about hearing aids by assessing three or more hearing aids in repeated measurement designs.

Independent Group Designs

Increasing the number of levels of the independent variable greatly increases the amount of information in independent group designs. In a study where the independent variable is language training and the dependent variable is scores on a language test, the results provide only one piece of information: children who are language disordered and receive language training score either higher, lower, or the same as children who do not receive training. If the independent variable has three levels—training by Method A, training by Method B, or no training, the results indicate whether either or both training methods are better than no training, and whether one training method is better than the other. More detailed information about the potential advantages of a training method can be obtained by comparing it with another method, as well as comparing it with no training.

Repeated Measurement Designs

Increasing the number of levels of the independent variable also gives more information in repeated measurement designs. A design that permits researchers to compare more than two hearing aids or more than two levels of background noise would greatly facilitate practical research.

As in the simple repeated measurement design, the effects of order of presentation must be controlled by counterbalancing. The more levels of the independent variable, the more complex the counterbalancing procedure. Each level has to occur at each position in the order an equal number of times. This can be done by complete counterbalancing, using all possible orders. However, the number of possible orders increases sharply with the number of levels of the independent variables. There are six possible orders for three levels, 24 for four levels and 120 for five levels.

An alternative is to use incomplete counterbalancing. The most common technique for incomplete counterbalancing is the *Latin Square*, where each level is presented once at each position in a given order of presentation. The Latin Squares in Table 6–1 could be used with three, four, and five levels of the independent variable, where the levels are labeled by letters.

TABLE 6–1.
Latin Squares Used with Three, Four, and Five Levels of an Independent Variable.

Order of Presentation	Levels of the Independent Variable											
	3			4				5				
1	A	B	C	A	B	C	D	A	B	C	D	E
2	B	C	A	D	C	B	A	E	D	B	C	A
3	C	A	B	C	A	D	B	D	C	A	E	B
4				B	D	A	C	C	A	E	B	D
5								B	E	D	A	C

Three subgroups of subjects would be needed to control for order effects with three levels, four with four levels and five with five levels of the independent variable. As in the simple repeated measurement design, counterbalancing serves as a control for the possible confounding of the independent variable by order effects. However, any order effects that did occur, such as practice effects, fatigue, or boredom, could become greater as the number of conditions increased. The increased variability associated with order effects could obscure the effect of the independent variable. Thus, counterbalancing controls for order effects but does not reduce them. It is best to plan a procedure that will minimize practice effects, fatigue, and boredom.

The possibility of more than two repeated measurements also increases the amount of information that can be obtained from training studies and other studies that assess performance over time. For example, assessment of vocabulary training would be more precise if several measures were obtained before, during, and after training. Assessment of the dependent variable several months or years after training has been completed is especially important for practical research. Multiple repeated measurements are also very useful in longitudinal studies where a dependent variable such as language ability is repeatedly measured over a number of years in HCD populations such as children who are language impaired and children who are hearing impaired.

FACTORIAL DESIGNS: MORE THAN
ONE INDEPENDENT VARIABLE

For many of the important problems of HCD research, simple research designs do not provide enough information. Even when the complexity of the design is increased by using more than two levels of the independent variable, more detailed information may be needed. Designs that vary two or more independent variables at the same time can provide detailed information suitable to the complexity of the processes and the disorders studied. Such designs are called *factorial designs*.

An important advantage of having more than one independent variable is that the characteristics of the populations can be better controlled. In studying the effect of training method on the language development of children who are hearing impaired, it is important to assess the effects of other independent variables at the same time. For example, both amount of hearing loss and duration of training have important effects on language acquisition. By varying amount of hearing loss and duration of training as additional independent variables, the effects of type of training can be determined more precisely. Language acquisition by the two training methods can be determined as a function of amount of hearing loss and duration of training. The methods may not be equally effective at each level of hearing impairment, and the course of language acquisition may differ for the two methods.

Another advantage of having more than one independent variable is that the characteristics of the communication processes studied can be better controlled. In acquired language disorders, it is likely that not all language abilities may be impaired to the same extent. To determine the characteristics of acquired language disorders more precisely, receptive versus expressive language could be one independent variable, and different levels of language (e.g., phonetic, phonological, lexical, syntactic, semantic, and pragmatic) could be a second independent variable. Language disorders might be most severe for one level of receptive language and for a different level of expressive language.

The example of acquired language disorders can also be used to illustrate the final advantage of studying more than one independent variable. The exact type of language disorder may vary as a function of the location of brain damage. To study the effects of both type and location of language disorder at the same time would require a factorial design that includes both independent groups and repeated measurements as independent variables. Such a design permits researchers to obtain more detailed information about complex populations and complex communication processes in the same design.

Factorial designs that include both independent groups and repeated measurements are called *mixed factorial designs*. In a mixed factorial design where the independent group variable is location of brain lesion and the repeated measurement variable is type of language disorder, the researchers might discover that the type of language disorder varies as a function of the location of the lesion. These results cannot be obtained with a simple design, or with an independent group or repeated measurement factorial design. Mixed independent group and repeated measurement factorial designs greatly extend the research capabilities of HCD researchers.

It might appear that HCD researchers can obtain precise information concerning all of the complexities of HCDs by using complex mixed factorial designs to study all relevant independent variables at the same time. Unfortunately, this is not the case. Complex factorial designs are very useful, but have their own particular limitations. The more complex the design, the greater the number of experimental conditions or *cells* in the factorial design. A design involving two independent variables with two levels each has four cells (2×2), a design with three independent variables with two levels each has eight cells ($2 \times 2 \times 2$), and a design that has four independent variables with five, four, three, and two levels, respectively, would have 120 cells. It is difficult to find enough subjects with the necessary characteristics to fill the cells of complex designs. For example, it would probably not be possible to find large enough subgroups of children who are hearing impaired to fill the cells of a design that varies type of training, amount of hearing impairment, and duration of training.

Interactions

As described previously, factorial designs provide more detailed information concerning gaps in knowledge than simple group designs. Not only can more independent variables be studied, but the relationships between the independent variables can be determined. Relationships are indicated by *interactions* between independent variables. In a 2×2 factorial design, if one independent variable has the same effect for both levels of the other independent variable, there is no interaction between the independent variables. If the first independent variable has one effect for one level and another effect for the other level of the second independent variable, there is an interaction. This sounds complicated, but a concrete example will illustrate the simplicity of such an interaction.

In a study using a 2×2 mixed factorial design, the independent group variable is left frontal lobe versus left temporal lobe brain lesions, the repeated measurement variable is receptive versus expressive language ability, and the dependent variable is scores on a test of receptive and expressive language ability. If both the frontal and the temporal lobe group were most impaired in expressive language, there would be no interaction between location of lesion and type of language impairment. For both groups, expressive language would be more impaired than receptive language. If the frontal lobe group was most impaired in expressive language, but the temporal lobe group was most impaired in receptive language, there would be an interaction between the location of lesion and the type of language impairment. The effect of frontal lobe lesions on language ability would be different than the effect of temporal lobe lesions. The information about interactions could be very useful for planning treatment.

One important advantage of factorial designs, then, is that they provide a way to determine whether the effects of one independent variable are the same for different levels of other independent variables. When the effects vary, they are described as interactions of independent variables. Other examples of interactions are given in this chapter, and also in Chapter 13.

SIMPLE FACTORIAL DESIGNS

The simplest factorial design has two independent variables, each with two levels, and is called a 2×2 factorial design. The numbers refer to the number of levels. A 2×2×2 factorial design has three independent variables, each with two levels, and a 3×4 factorial design has two independent variables, one with three levels and the other with four levels.

The two independent variables in the simple 2×2 design can both be independent groups, both repeated measures, or one independent group and one repeated measure. Examples of these simple designs will make it much easier to understand the more complex factorial designs.

2×2 Independent Group Designs

The 2×2 independent group design could be used in HCD research when one independent variable is a natural group difference between HCD and normal subjects and the other is a natural group difference that would provide more detailed information about the HCD. In a study of higher-order language skills in children with articulation/phonological disorders versus normal children, more detailed information would be obtained with sex as a second independent variable. If the difference in language ability between children who are articulation disordered and children who are not was the same for girls and boys, there would be no interaction between sex and articulation disorders. If the difference in language ability between children who are articulation disordered and children who are not was larger for boys, there would be an interaction. With this particular example, further research might be needed before practical application. To obtain more insight about the difference between sexes, age might be added as a third independent variable in further research.

2×2 Repeated Measurement Designs

In studies of the effect of two different treatments on a group with HCD, it may be useful to assess the treatments in different situations. In comparing word recognition by adults with conductive hearing loss for two different hearing aids, word recognition could be measured in a quiet situation and a noisy situation. The two independent variables would be hearing aids and noise, each with two levels. The resulting comparison would provide very useful information. There might be no difference between aids in quiet, but one aid might improve word recognition more in noise. It would seem best to choose an aid that worked best in noise.

If, however, one aid was found to be better in quiet and the other in noise, patients who needed to hear in quiet would choose one aid and those who needed to hear in noisy conditions would choose the other aid. Those who could afford two aids could use one aid in quiet and the other in noise. The discovery of an interaction between the repeated measurement variables of noise level and hearing aid effectiveness could have very important implications for hearing aid users.

In factorial as well as simple repeated measurement designs it is necessary to control for order of presentation by counterbalancing. In the previous example, at least four subgroups of subjects would be needed. The four orders of presentation could be counterbalanced by a Latin Square procedure, as described previously.

2×2 Mixed Designs

The mixed factorial design that uses both independent groups and repeated measurements is very common in HCD research. In the preceding chapter, two different research designs were suggested for studying the effects of vocabulary training on children who are language impaired. The random selection design compared a trained and an untrained group. The repeated measurement design compared vocabulary scores before and after training for one group. More complete information about the effects of training could be obtained by combining the two designs into a 2×2 mixed design. In the mixed design, the independent group variable would be training versus no training and the repeated measurement independent variable would be time of testing. If the groups were similar in vocabulary before training, but the trained group had a much larger vocabulary after training, the interaction between training and time of testing would demonstrate the effectiveness of training.

The mixed factorial design overcomes the limitations of the two simple designs. The use of two independent variables would eliminate the possible effects of uncontrolled variables in the simple independent group design and the possible practice, fatigue, or boredom effects in the simple repeated measurement design.

COMPLEX FACTORIAL DESIGNS

The simplest factorial design is the 2×2 design with two levels of two independent variables that may be independent groups, repeated measurements, or both. Factorial designs can be made more complex by increasing the number of independent variables, the number of levels of independent variables, or both. There can be three or more independent variables, and three or more levels of each independent variable. Thus, the complexity of the design can be increased to equal the complexity of the process studied. Several examples will illustrate the usefulness of complex factorial designs for HCD research.

If researchers wished to study the effects of linguistic complexity on stuttering, their present knowledge of stuttering might suggest the importance of determining the effects of linguistic complexity separately for subjects of different sexes and amounts of education. This could be accomplished by a factorial design that had three independent variables with two levels each, a 2×2×2 factorial design, as shown in Table 6–2.

TABLE 6–2.
A 2×2×2 Factorial Design.

Independent Variables	Levels	
Linguistic complexity	Simple vs. Complex	Repeated Measurement
Sex	Male vs. Female	Independent Groups
Education	High School vs. University	Independent Groups

The linguistic complexity variable would be a repeated measurement and the other independent variables would be independent groups. The dependent variable would be amount of nonfluency on an oral reading task that included simple and complex passages presented in counterbalanced order.

Complex factorial designs are interpreted in the same manner as simple factorial designs, but there are many more possible outcomes. In the present example, the basic interest is in the effects of the independent variable of linguistic complexity on the dependent variable of nonfluency. Are there more nonfluencies on complex than on simple oral reading passages? This question could be answered by use of a simple repeated measures design with the independent variable being two repeated measurements for one group. The complex factorial design provides more detailed information about different subgroups.

If the total group is less fluent when reading complex passages, does this complexity effect occur to the same extent in subjects of different sexes and amounts of education? It might be found that the complexity effect is greater for male subjects than for female subjects, and greater for high school than for university subjects. These would be *simple interactions* between the complexity effect and each of the other independent variables. The complex factorial design would provide a great deal more information than the simple design. The finding that the effects of linguistic complexity on stuttering vary as a function of both sex and education could be very useful information for the practitioner.

However, the complex factorial design can yield still more information in the form of *complex interactions*. Such interactions are often considered too difficult to interpret, but there is no difficulty if the logic used to interpret simple interactions is applied to the complex interactions. For the simple interactions, the question was whether the same complexity effect occurred for subjects of different sexes and different education levels. For the more complex interaction, one question is whether the interaction between complexity and education level is the same for male and female subjects. The complexity effect might occur for both high school and university male subjects, but only for high school female subjects. This interaction between linguistic complexity, sex, and education could also provide useful information for the practitioner. The joint effects of sex and education could dictate different treatment strategies for female subjects but not for male subjects as a function of their education.

Practitioners might feel that even more information should be obtained by increasing the number of levels of independent variables. Three or four levels of linguistic complexity and three or four levels of education might be more informative. Additional independent variables might also provide more useful information. The practitioner might be concerned with linguistic complexity effects before and after treatment. If the effects of different types of treatment were also of interest, still another independent variable would be added.

Very detailed information about a problem can be obtained by using the factorial design strategy of selecting independent variables of interest and varying the number of levels of each independent variable as needed. The limitations of complex factorial designs are the numbers of subjects and experimental conditions required by the design. This depends on the number of cells in the design. The number of cells is calculated by multiplying the number of levels for each independent variable. Where there are the three independent variables of linguistic complexity, sex, and education with two levels each, there is a $2 \times 2 \times 2$ factorial design with eight cells. The eight cells would consist of two repeated measurement cells for each of four groups. The four groups are high school male, high school female, university male, and university female subjects.

If the levels of complexity were increased to three and the levels of education to four, the design would become a $3 \times 2 \times 4$ factorial design with three repeated measurement cells for each of eight groups. If the number of independent variables was increased by varying the type of reading passage with three levels (fiction, nonfiction, and poetry) and the type of treatment with three levels (behavioral, psychoanalytic, and combined), the design would become a $3 \times 3 \times 2 \times 4 \times 3$ factorial design with nine repeated measurement cells for each of 24 groups.

As this example indicates, increasing the complexity of the design would soon result in too many experimental conditions and groups. Complex factorial designs can provide very detailed information. Such information may be useful for planning different types of treatment for different types of clients in different communication situations. However, the number and the levels of independent variables must be selected with the greatest of care to avoid designing a study with too many groups of subjects and experimental conditions.

NUMBER OF SUBJECTS NEEDED FOR COMPLEX GROUP DESIGNS

The reasoning used in deciding on the number of subjects needed for complex group designs is the same as that used for simple group designs. The larger the expected treatment effects and the smaller the within-group variance, the fewer subects are needed. Preliminary information about these values is helpful. In the absence of such information, a very rough estimate of the minimum number of subjects is 5 to 10 subjects per independent group or repeated measurement cell. For example, a minimum of 20 to 40 subjects would be needed for the four cells of a 2×2 factorial design and a minimum of 300 to 600 subjects for the 60 cells of a $3 \times 4 \times 5$ factorial design.

COMPLEX CORRELATION DESIGNS

Simple correlation designs provide information about the relationship between two variables such as language ability and reading achievement in children who are hearing impaired. Like simple independent group or repeated measurement designs, simple correlation designs may not provide enough information. Complex correlation designs provide more information about relationships. These designs are usually considered statistical techniques rather than research designs. They are discussed here as research designs, as they provide additional ways of obtaining information about HCDs. The number of subjects required for complex correlations is an important consideration. A very rough estimate of the minimum number is 10 to 20 subjects per variable correlated.

Partial Correlation

Where other variables affect the relationship between two variables, their effects can be controlled by a *partial correlation* design. For example, in studying the relationship between language ability and reading achievement in children who are hearing impaired, it might not be possible to test all children of the same age or to control age by testing different age groups. Both reading and language ability should increase with age. If age effects were not controlled, the correlation between language ability and reading achievement could be confounded by their joint relationship with age. In such a case, the effects of age could be held constant by partial correlation, which would adjust the correlation between language ability and reading achievement to eliminate the effects of their correlation with age.

Multiple Correlation

When there is need to determine the relationship between one variable and a number of other variables operating jointly, the multiple correlation between the *criterion variables* and the *predictor variable* can be determined. For example, it may be useful to assess the relationship between different levels of language ability and reading achievement. The joint relationship of phonetic, phonological, lexical, syntactic, and semantic ability to reading achievement would be determined by *multiple correlation*.

Multiple Regression

Multiple regression designs go one step further than multiple correlation designs. They provide information about the unique relationship between each predictor variable and the criterion variable. This useful information cannot be obtained from separate correlations between criterion variable and each of the predictor variables. It is necessary to control for the correlations between the different predictor variables by multiple regression. Multiple regression thus combines the functions of partial correlation and multiple correlation.

The multiple regression design would appear to be an ideal method for finding the causes of HCDs. By means of the multiple regression design, the independent correlations between predictor (possible causal) variables and the criterion variable (HCD) could be determined. However, there are limitations to the application of multiple regression designs to HCD research. The demonstration of a relationship between variables is not sufficient to prove that changes in one variable cause changes in the other variable; and the more variables that are correlated, the more subjects are needed.

Factor Analysis and Cluster Analysis

Factor analysis is a correlation design that groups variables together on the basis of their interrelationships. In a study of the pattern of language deficit associated with childhood language disorders, a large number of language measures might be obtained in a preliminary study. The number of measures could be reduced by factor analysis without reducing the range of abilities assessed. Factor analysis groups measures that are highly correlated with each other into factors that are independent of each other. Then a single measure that best represents each factor can be selected.

After a preliminary factor analysis of the language abilities of normal children, children with language disorders could be compared to children with normal language by using only one measure for each of the independent factors. The information could be obtained more rapidly, avoiding boredom and fatigue from taking all of the original tests, and the resulting pattern of deficit would be more easy to interpret.

Another form of factor analysis called the *Q-technique of factor analysis* is also useful for HCD research. With the Q-technique, subjects are grouped together on the basis of the similarity in their patterns of test scores. If a battery of language tests is given to a group of children with language disorders, the children will be grouped into "factors" by the Q-technique. Children with one pattern of language deficit will be grouped into one factor and children with other patterns will be grouped into other factors. For example, children with particular difficulty on tests of language comprehension might be grouped together in a factor designated as receptive language disorder, and children with particular difficulty on tests of language production might be grouped together into a factor designated as expressive language disorder. Such groupings of children into language disorder subtypes could have important implications for intervention.

Cluster analysis is another method for grouping subjects on the basis of patterns of deficit. The correlational design is the same as the Q-technique of factor analysis, but the mathematical procedures for grouping subjects are different.

COMBINED CORRELATION AND GROUP DESIGNS

For certain purposes it is advantageous to combine correlation and group designs. Three types of combined design that have been used in HCD research are *covariance designs*, *multivariate designs*, and *discriminant analysis designs*.

Covariance Designs

In group designs where it is difficult to control variables that might influence the independent variables, a covariance design can be used to hold the effects of the variable constant. Covariance designs are statistical control procedures that serve a function similar to partial correlation. In a study that compares the language abilities of normal children and children with cerebral palsy, it might be difficult to match the groups in age. The covariance design would adjust the language scores of the groups to compensate for the difference in age. This design can be considered an alternative to matched group designs.

Multivariate Designs

All of the simple and complex group designs discussed so far have only one dependent variable. Studies with more than one dependent variable are called multivariate designs. The multivariate design controls for the correlations between dependent variables. If researchers wanted to assess the effects of a treatment method on a variety of behaviors, they could use a multivariate design to compared treated and nontreated groups. The effects of the independent variables can be determined for all dependent variables acting together, and for each dependent variable separately.

Discriminant Analysis Designs

Where the object of a study is to obtain a measure that will best differentiate two or more HCD groups from each other or from a normal control group, a number of variables on which the groups differ can be measured. Then a statistical procedure called discriminant analysis is performed to calculate a combined *weighted score* for all the measures that best differentiate the groups. For example, a number of measures of lip, tongue, and jaw movement might be obtained in a large group of babies. The measures would be used in a discriminant analysis several years later to compare children who developed articulation/phonological disorders with normally speaking children. The proportion that each measure contributed to the total weighted score would be varied until the weighted score that best differentiated the two groups was found. This score could be used to predict which babies are most likely to develop articulation disorders. Like other complex designs, a limitation of this design is that the more variables are measured, the more subjects are needed.

ADDITIONAL INFORMATION

Additional information about complex factorial designs can be found in Shaughnessy and Zechmeister (1985) and the other texts listed in Chapter 5; information about correlation designs can be found in Edwards (1984) and Pedhazur and Kerlinger (1982) and other advanced statistics texts; and information about combined correlation and group designs can be found in Tabachnick and Fidell (1983) and other advanced statistics texts.

REVIEW QUESTIONS

1. In what ways may complex group designs differ from simple group designs?
2. List the complex group designs discussed in this chapter.
3. What are the minimum number of subjects required for factorial designs and correlation designs?
4. What is an interaction? Give three examples of interactions that might occur in 2×2 factorial designs.
5. What are the practical limitations of factorial designs?
6. Briefly state the purpose of each of the complex correlation designs and the combined correlation and group designs.

EXERCISES (answers are given in Appendix D)

1. For each of the following problems:
Tell what kind of complex group design (not including complex correlation designs or combined correlation and group designs) is most appropriate (e.g., independent group design with more than two levels of the independent variable, mixed 2×2 factorial design).
Give the independent variable(s), levels of each independent variable, dependent variable, and minimum number of subjects.
Indicate counterbalancing requirements.
Finally, for factorial designs, give an example of an interaction that might occur for that particular problem.

a. What is the effect of background noise on the recognition of words presented in isolation and words presented in sentences?
b. What effect does age have on speech perception?
c. What is the effect of voice disorders on the speech intelligibility of male and female subjects?
d. What is the effect of different amounts of background noise on speech perception?
e. Do voice disorders affect vowels more than consonants?

CHAPTER

7

Advantages and Disadvantages of Group Research Designs

The group research designs described in Chapters 5 and 6 provide researchers with many different ways for obtaining information about HCDs. The levels of an independent variable, the number of independent variables, and the number of dependent variables can be adjusted by the designer to meet the requirements of particular research problems. Factorial designs permit the precise analysis of interactions between independent variables, enabling researchers to determine the complex relationships that exist among variables affecting HCDs. Further information about relationships can be obtained by the use of correlation designs and designs that combine correlation and factorial designs.

Although group research designs are often used, they do not meet all of the needs of HCD research. Information about HCDs can be obtained in other ways by other types of research design. HCD researchers should know when to use standard group designs and when to use other designs. No design is ideal for all problems that concern HCD researchers—each has its strengths and weaknesses.

Before the other designs are described in the next chapter, the advantages and disadvantages of group designs for HCD research will be summarized here. Then the advantages and disadvantages of other research designs can be related to those of group designs. These distinctions are important, because there is a natural tendency to adopt one type of design for all purposes. HCD researchers should be aware of the advantages and disadvantages of all research designs. This knowledge will help them to choose the designs most appropriate for the problems they wish to study, and to obtain information of most use to practitioners.

ADVANTAGES OF GROUP RESEARCH DESIGNS

Group designs were developed to isolate the effects of independent variables, control the effects of other variables, obtain detailed information about interactions between independent variables, demonstrate causal relationships, and generalize findings. Where designs are successful in achieving some or all of these purposes, useful information about HCDs can be obtained.

Isolating the Effects of Independent Variables

Group designs systematically vary the levels of independent variables to determine the effects on dependent variables. Independent variables can be groups of subjects, or repeated measurements of the same subjects, or both.

Controlling the Effects of Other Variables

Variables other than the independent variables might affect dependent variables, and thus, confound the effects of the independent variables. Group designs control the effects of other variables by allowing them to vary randomly in random selection designs, by holding them constant in matched group designs, or by systematically varying them in factorial designs.

Obtaining Detailed Information about Interactions

Factorial designs provide information about how the effect of an independent variable on a dependent variable may change as a function of changes in other independent variables. Such designs have proved very useful for studying the complexities of HCDs and for obtaining the type of detailed information needed for practical applications of research findings.

Generalizing Findings

A basic purpose of group designs is to generalize information from samples of subjects to the populations from which the subjects were obtained. The conditions necessary for generalization to entire populations are seldom met, because entire populations are seldom available for HCD research. However, limited generalizations are possible in group designs. This is an important advantage, as generalization is difficult with other designs.

Demonstrating Causal Relationships

When the necessary conditions for causal inferences have been met, group designs can lead to an understanding of the phenomena. Shaughnessy and Zechmeister (1985, pp. 23–25) have described three conditions that must be met in group designs to permit causal inferences. A change in the independent variable must be accompanied by a change in the dependent variable, the change in the independent variable must precede the change in the dependent variable, and plausible alternative causes must be eliminated. The third condition is met by controlling relevant variables or allowing them to vary randomly. These conditions are easiest to meet with random selection, random assignment, and matched group designs where the independent variable is training.

DISADVANTAGES OF GROUP RESEARCH DESIGNS

Group designs have been borrowed from psychological research, where their function is to arrive at a basic understanding of human behavior. Such designs may not be completely suitable for all HCD research problems. The main disadvantages of group research designs for HCD research are difficulty in meeting the requirements of group designs, limitations of information about groups, limitations of quantitative information, inapplicability to practical settings, and difficulty in proving cause-and-effect relationships. These disadvantages will be discussed separately.

Difficulty in Meeting the Requirements of Group Designs

Under ideal circumstances, groups are randomly sampled from the populations being studied. Situation variables that might affect the independent variables under study are held constant or systematically varied.

Information about dependent variables obtained under these highly controlled conditions isolates the effects of the independent variables.

These ideal conditions can seldom be met in HCD research. Matched groups and natural groups are used instead of randomly selected groups, and relevant variables cannot be completely controlled. Relevant variables can be controlled to some extent by making them independent variables in complex factorial designs. However, such designs often require more groups than are available to HCD researchers.

Compromises in ideal group designs are unavoidable. Matched groups and natural groups are used instead of random groups. Not all relevant variables are completely controlled. Because of the difficulty of obtaining large numbers of subjects with the desired characteristics, groups may be very small, and the number and the levels of independent variables may be restricted. Such restrictions limit the interpretations of results obtained with group designs and decrease the knowledge that can be obtained with these designs. HCD researchers who use group designs must guard against the tendency to interpret their findings as though they had met all the requirements of random group designs.

Limitations of Information about Groups

Even when the ideal requirements of group designs can be met, the information obtained applies only to the group as a whole, not to individuals. To the extent that the trends for each individual are the same as the group average, the information can be of practical use. Where there are large differences between individuals, group averages may not adequately represent the characteristics of individuals, and the information may not be useful for practical applications.

Limitations of Quantitative Information

In group designs, the dependent variables are expressed as numerical quantities to permit statements about the probability of the effects of the independent variables. Even when the requirements of group designs have been met and group results adequately represent individual performance, a quantified measure of the dependent variable may not provide enough information. The desired information about HCDs may be difficult to express in numerical form. For example, the operations of the speech mechanism involve complex movements that cannot be easily described in quantitative form, and a single numerical score may not adequately represent complex processes such as syntactic ability.

Inapplicability to Natural Communication Situations

Group designs control the research environment to isolate the effects of independent variables. Information about persons with HCDs obtained under such conditions may not indicate how they will perform in natural situations. The term *ecological validity* is sometimes used in addition to the term *external validity* to describe the need for experimental findings to apply to natural settings.

The problem of ecological validity is greater for some aspects of HCDs than for others. For disorders such as conductive hearing loss, information obtained in the controlled situations required by group designs may apply to natural settings. However, information obtained under controlled conditions about disorders such as stuttering may not apply to natural settings.

Ecological validity can also be a problem in clinical practice. Changes in HCDs in the controlled clinic setting may not carry over to the natural communication situation. Clinical methods have been developed to facilitate carry-over from the clinic to the natural setting. Whenever possible, researchers should attempt to assess carry-over from the research situation to natural settings.

Identification of Causes

It is difficult to meet all three conditions for causal inference with the use of group designs for HCD research. The first condition can be met when a change in the independent variable (the causal variable) is associated with a change in the dependent variable.

The second condition is met in designs where an experimental treatment such as vocabulary training is applied, and the dependent variable changes after the treatment has been applied. However, much HCD research involves the measurement of existing variables rather than the measurement of changes resulting from experimental treatments, and in such research causal inferences are not possible.

The third condition is met when all variables that might affect the dependent variable are controlled in order to rule out the possibility that changes in uncontrolled variables caused changes in the dependent variable. This condition can be met only by random group and matched group designs. With natural groups, the possibility that some uncontrolled variables may affect the dependent variable cannot be ruled out.

Designs that do not meet all three conditions can only prove that independent and dependent variables are related, not that changes in independent variables cause changes in dependent variables. Studies that do not meet all three conditions are called *correlational studies* to distinguish them from studies of causal relationships. This is somewhat confusing, because correlation designs are different from group designs. However, the use of the term *correlational* does indicate that certain group designs do not permit causal inferences.

CONCLUSIONS

HCD research would be much easier if a few group designs met all needs. However, a variety of group designs and other designs are required. Researchers who use group designs without recognizing their limitations are likely to misinterpret their findings, to the detriment of persons with HCDs. Researchers who reject group designs because of their limitations may fail to use the most appropriate design, also to the detriment of persons with HCDs. Awareness of the advantages and disadvantages of group designs provides a basis for evaluating the advantages and disadvantages of the remaining designs discussed in the next chapter.

ADDITIONAL INFORMATION

The advantages and disadvantages of group designs are discussed in most texts on research design, such as those listed at the end of Chapters 4 and 5. Detail concerning limitations of group designs can be found in Cook and Campbell (1979), with the first chapter devoted to causal inference. Many books on qualitative methodology begin with a discussion of the limitations of group designs, but usually do not pay as much attention to the advantages of group designs.

REVIEW QUESTIONS

1. List and briefly describe the advantages and disadvantages of group designs.
2. Discuss the reasons why researchers should not completely accept or completely reject group designs.

CHAPTER

8

Other Research Designs

HCD researchers may decide to use research designs other than standard group research designs for a number of reasons, as discussed in previous chapters. There may not be enough subjects available to meet the requirements of the group research design appropriate for their problem. They may wish to obtain information about individuals rather than groups, information that cannot be expressed in the quantitative form required for group designs, or information in natural situations rather than controlled experimental settings. Finally, they may be studying aspects of HCDs that are so regular that group studies are unnecessary. Other research designs that might be selected in such circumstances are described in this chapter.

The research designs discussed here include observation in natural settings, case studies, descriptive methods, single-subject designs, quasi-experimental designs for research in natural settings, and qualitative methods. These designs fulfill needs that are not met by standard group designs. They may lack some of the advantages of group designs for isolating the effects of independent variables, controlling the effects of other variables, obtaining detailed information about interactions, demonstrating causal relationships, and generalizing findings. However, it is important to be aware of these alternative designs. HCD research is becoming concerned with the more subtle, context-dependent aspects of communication. Standard group designs may not provide the most appropriate means of investigating such phenomena.

OBSERVATION IN NATURAL SETTINGS

Observational methods differ from standard group designs in several ways. Quantitative or qualitative information about individuals is obtained in natural settings. There is no attempt to control all relevant variables in order to isolate the effects of independent variables. However, observational methods should not be confused with the casual observations made in everyday life. The behaviors to be observed are defined in advance, and the observations are carefully recorded. The objective is to identify relationships among variables in natural contexts. In some cases, it is the effect of the context that is being studied.

Several variations of observational methods are available to HCD researchers. These involve different degrees of intervention in the situation by the observers. Different types of data can be recorded from observational research, ranging from complete descriptions of the events observed to the recording of specific units of behavior. Several types of observation method will be briefly described as related to HCD research (see Shaughnessy & Zechmeister [1985] for more complete descriptions).

Observation without Intervention

The observation method most different from standard group designs is *observation without intervention*, where there are passive observers who simply record the events that occur in natural settings. These methods are also called *naturalistic observation* or *naturalistic field studies*. The goal is to observe behavior as it occurs in natural settings. In HCD research, naturalistic observation can be used to verify relationships among variables found by the use of standard group designs. For example, HCD and non-HCD subjects could be observed in natural settings to verify differences in characteristics such as misarticulation, voice disorders, or nonfluency, and to determine whether special training results in improved communication in natural settings. Naturalistic observation can also be used to determine the effects of different contexts on HCDs, for example, whether the rate of dysfluency varies in home, school, recreational, and vocational settings.

Observation with Intervention

To obtain particular types of information, observers may intervene in several different ways. In *participant observation* the observer becomes a participant in the situation in order to understand the situation of the person observed. To better understand the effects of hearing impairment, a participant observer might live with the family of a child who is hearing impaired for a period of time. In *structured observation* the observers control the situation in certain ways to obtain the desired information. A child with language disorder and a child without language disorder might be put in a play situation with specially selected toys to learn about the communicative interactions of children with language disorders in natural settings. More situational control is exerted in *field experiments*, where an elaborate situation may be "staged" to determine its effects on participants. Stutterers might be asked to participate in situations where the other participants have been trained to exhibit anger, impatience, scorn, and sympathy, to determine the effects of such social stresses on dysfluency.

Communicative Interactions

A type of structured observation that is used very often in HCD research is the observation of communicative interactions in natural settings. The communicative interactions usually involve various combinations of children with and without HCDs, and children interacting with adults. These structured observations often provide the best way of obtaining the desired information about the effects of HCDs. They are of special interest with regard to research design, because what is observed is an interaction between two or more subjects, not the response of a subject to a controlled stimulus. The researchers usually have to reach conclusions concerning the HCDs of one of the participants. The observations are seldom entirely naturalistic. Units of communicative behavior are defined in advance, and are selectively observed. The resulting data can be analyzed by quantitative methods.

Advantages and Disadvantages of Observational Methods

Advantages of observational methods are that the setting is much closer to real-life settings and clinic settings, and observations are not necessarily restricted to quantitative measurements of a small set of variables. Disadvantages are that the information obtained from observations of individuals in particular natural settings cannot easily be generalized to others with HCDs or to all situations, and the lack of systematic control of relevant variables does not provide precise information about interactions, correlations, or causal relationships.

Problems that researchers must be particularly concerned with in natural observation are observer bias and subject bias. Researchers must rule out the possibility that observers will be unduly influenced by what they expect and hope to observe, and the possibility that the subjects will be unduly influenced by the knowledge that they are being observed.

Researchers may choose observational methods instead of group designs because no group designs are suitable for studying communicative interactions and other complex events. Another important reason for using observational methods is to generate hypotheses about HCDs that can be studied under more controlled conditions in further research. Observational methods provide detailed, ecologically valid information that cannot be obtained in any other way. They are valuable tools for HCD researchers.

CASE STUDIES

The classic method for obtaining detailed information about individuals with HCDs is the case study. The information can be obtained from a number of sources, including developmental history, medical history, home and educational background, clinical observations, test results, and responses to treatment. Case studies may be restricted to one individual with a rare disorder, or to a series of individuals with similar disorders. They can be used to supplement the information obtained from group designs. The case study method is especially appropriate for obtaining information about types of HCD that occur too rarely to be studied by group designs. For example, there are relatively few deaf-blind individuals, but it is important to evaluate the effectiveness of communicative training. This is better done by case studies than by group designs.

A major advantage of case studies is that there is no restriction on the amount or type of information included. In addition, they can suggest directions for further research, they can be used to study new techniques and rare phenomena, and they can provide important tests for theories. The disadvantages are that it is difficult to generalize from a single case, uncontrolled observations of individuals do not provide information about interactions, correlations, or causal relationships, and there can be bias in the selection of cases, the selection of information about cases, and the interpretation of findings.

Researchers may do case studies when other designs are inappropriate, or to obtain information for planning research that uses other designs. Conclusions from case studies are informed guesswork. Practitioners who keep detailed case histories concerning particularly informative cases can present their findings as case studies. Thus, the case study brings researchers and practitioners close together.

INDIVIDUAL DESCRIPTION

Some HCDs involve uniform physiological processes. When variability between individuals is small enough, group designs are unnecessary. Useful information can be obtained by observation of individuals under carefully controlled conditions. Examples would be studies of reflex responses of jaw, lip, and tongue muscles. Where individual differences in uncontrolled variables do not confound the effects of independent variables, the findings of individual descriptive studies can be generalized to others in the same population. Where the level of the independent variable is changed as part of the study, information can be obtained about cause-and-effect relationships, as in the effect of cleft palate surgery on speech. For certain phenomena, then, the objectives of group designs can be achieved in descriptive studies of individuals. It is important for HCD researchers to be aware of this possibility, even though such phenomena may be relatively rare.

GROUP DESCRIPTION

HCD research sometimes involves very careful studies that do not determine the effects of independent variables, but simply describe variables of interest in a normal population or a population with HCD. The information is obtained under the carefully controlled conditions that are required by group designs, but there is no experiment. The results are reported in detail to provide information about the range of variation in normal or HCD populations. For example, spontaneous speech samples might be obtained for a large sample of normal speakers to determine the incidence of dysfluencies in normal speech. Another example of group description designs would be surveys of a population through questionnaires. Surveys can reveal important information about the characteristics, attitudes, educational achievements, and case histories of large samples of HCDs. However, there may be questions about the reliability of self reports. Group descriptions can provide information of use to both practitioners and researchers.

SINGLE-SUBJECT RESEARCH DESIGNS

Operant conditioning methods devised by B. F. Skinner and his associates to study animal behavior have been adapted to study the behavior of individual subjects under highly controlled conditions. Where these *single-subject designs* can be applied, group designs may not be needed to demonstrate causal relationships.

Single-subject designs may be used to assess the effects of treatment or training. They are comparable to random selection group designs where the independent variable is treatment or training. As compared with natural observation, the experimental situation is very carefully controlled. Relevant variables are held constant or systematically varied to permit the determination of causal relationships between the independent and dependent variables. The conclusions are based on many observations under very specific conditions.

In HCD research, single-subject designs can be used to evaluate methods for improving communication skills or for eliminating impairments that impede communication. For example, they may be used to teach speech, hearing, and language skills to children who are hearing impaired, to help aphasic patients recover language skills, and to reduce dysfluencies in stutterers. The researcher always begins by determining a *baseline* for the behavior that is to be changed. Enough measures are taken that a confident statement can be made concerning the stability of pretreatment dependent variables such as misarticulations of children who are hearing impaired, word-finding difficulties of aphasic patients, or dysfluencies of stutterers.

When the baseline has been established, the treatment is applied until the *target behavior* changes. The treatment is a procedure that can be repeatedly applied, such as word repetition, picture naming, or speech timed by a metronome. Correct responses are rewarded according to a schedule of reinforcement. Other situational variables are carefully controlled. A change in the target behavior after a single treatment is not sufficient proof of a causal relationship between the treatment and the target behavior. There are several procedures for obtaining sufficient proof, which will be described here. More complete details regarding the use of single-subject designs in HCD research can be found in McReynolds and Kearns (1983).

Withdrawal and Reversal Designs

The ideal single-subject designs are withdrawal and reversal designs. After several baseline measures, a treatment is given until the target behavior changes. Then the treatment is taken away (withdrawal design) or non-target behaviors are reinforced (reversal design) until the target behavior returns to baseline. This procedure proves that the treatment caused the change in behavior. When there is baseline, treatment, and either withdrawal or reversal, it is an ABA design. When the treatment is given again after withdrawal or reversal, it is an ABAB design, which provides more complete proof of the effectiveness of treatment. These designs can only be used in HCD research where treatment effects may be temporary rather than permanent, such as temporary decreases in the rate of dysfluencies of stutterers.

The Multiple Baseline Design

Another way to demonstrate the effect of a treatment is the multiple baseline design. Treatment effects are first demonstrated for one dependent variable, and then for one or more additional dependent variables. For example, in teaching children to articulate phonemes, one phoneme can be trained as the target behavior and two other phonemes can be assessed as nontarget baselines. If the first phoneme is trained and the nontarget baselines do not change, then a nontarget phoneme can be trained and compared with the remaining nontarget baseline. This multiple baseline procedure is not appropriate if there is generalization from the trained target behavior to nontrained nontarget behaviors, that is, if training a child to articulate one speech sound results in a change in the baselines for the other speech sounds.

There are several variations of the multiple baseline design. One is to establish a baseline for several subjects and then introduce the treatment at different times for the different subjects. If the baseline behavior changes only when the treatment is introduced, there is evidence of a causal relationship.

Other Single-Subject Designs

Where withdrawal, reversal, and multiple baseline designs cannot be used, a number of additional designs are available. As is the case for group designs, there is one ideal design—the withdrawal or reversal design—and all others sacrifice some of the rigorous controls afforded by this design.

Advantages and Disadvantages of Single-Subject Designs

Single-subject designs have some of the advantages of group designs and some of the advantages of observational and case study designs. Experimental conditions are rigorously controlled to obtain information about causal relationships between independent and dependent variables. Large groups of subjects are not needed, as information is obtained for individuals rather than groups. The information may have direct practical applications.

Single-subject designs also have disadvantages. Stable baselines may be difficult to establish for certain behaviors. Reversal designs cannot be used where treatment effects do not reverse, and multiple baseline designs cannot be used where treatment effects generalize to nontreated behaviors.

The very rigid control procedures may make the treatment too artificial for direct application by practitioners. The treatment may change the target behaviors only in the experimental situation and not in natural communication situations. If the treatment is not immediately effective in changing the baseline behavior, it may be difficult to demonstrate causal relationships. Finally, there is the same problem as in observation and case studies, a difficulty in generalizing the results. There is no way of predicting that all subjects of the same type will show the same treatment effects. Informed guesswork is unavoidable in interpreting the results of single-subject research.

HCD researchers should always keep single-subject designs in mind when planning research for which it is necessary to demonstrate causal relationships. Some of the limitations of these designs may be overcome by using them in combination with other designs.

QUASI-EXPERIMENTAL DESIGNS FOR RESEARCH IN NATURAL SETTINGS

As discussed in Chapter 7, it is difficult to demonstrate causal relationships by using standard group designs for HCD research. Research that demonstrates causal relationships can have great practical importance. There is no other way to prove that treatments are effective. Single-subject designs can be used to demonstrate causal relationships, but may not be appropriate for evaluating the benefits of treatments in natural settings. Research designs called *quasi-experimental designs* have been developed to provide information about causal relationships in natural settings. These designs attempt to control as many as possible of the variables that are difficult to control in natural settings. Some of the most common quasi-experimental designs will be described here. Others may be found in the reference sources listed at the end of the chapter.

Nonequivalent Control Group Designs

Nonequivalent control group designs are intended to control variables that might confound the effects of treatment in an experimental treatment group. They are similar to natural group designs as used in treatment studies, except that there is less control of relevant variables. An intact group such as a group of hearing impaired adults who receive auditory training together are compared with another intact group such as a group of adults who are hearing impaired and have not yet begun training. The groups are compared on a pre- and posttraining measure such as speech-reading ability. Relevant variables such as age, sex, amount of hearing loss, and education are not controlled. Special measures are needed to guard against the "Hawthorne effect," that is, a change resulting from the special attention received by the experimental group rather than from the exact type of training.

Interrupted Time Series Designs

Interrupted time-series designs are intended to rule out the possible effects of other variables at the exact time that the treatment was introduced. They are similar to ABA single-subject designs, as carried out in natural settings. The dependent variable is assessed a number of times before and after a treatment is given. If a group of hearing impaired adults is to be given auditory training, their speechreading abilities are assessed on a number of occasions before and after a period of intensive auditory training. Conclusions regarding a cause-and-effect relationship between training and speechreading ability depend on the degree of confidence that something else did not happen at the same time as auditory training to improve speechreading. As in the nonequivalent control group design, there is need to guard against the Hawthorne effect.

Combined Nonequivalent Control Group and Interrupted Time Series Design

Better evidence of causal relationships may be obtained by using a design that combines the nonequivalent control group and time-series designs. Both a trained and an untrained group would be tested a number of times before auditory training was given to the trained group. This combined design would further isolate the effects of the independent variable, controlling both for the occurrence and the timing of treatment. Once again, there is a need to guard against the Hawthorne effect.

Passive Observation Designs

A number of designs are available to evaluate naturally occurring causal relationships that do not involve special treatments. This is done by "passive observation" of causal relationships between variables measured on several occasions over a period of time. For example, a causal relationship between rubella during pregnancy and congenital sensorineural hearing impairment could be inferred by correlating the occurrence or nonoccurrence of rubella in the mother with the subsequent occurrence or nonoccurrence of sensorineural impairment in the child. Passive observation designs include *causal path analysis, cross-lagged panel correlations*, and *causal analysis of concomitancies in time series*. The choice of method depends on the types of events that are passively observed. These designs do not eliminate all of the problems of inferring causality from correlations. It is recommended that they be used to obtain preliminary information, and followed up by further research.

Advantages and Disadvantages of Quasi-Experimental Designs

Quasi-experimental designs are attempts to overcome the difficulties of applying group designs to research on causal relationships in natural settings. They are used only when random group designs are not appropriate. They are intended to go as far as possible toward determining causal relationships in natural settings, but must always be interpreted with great caution regarding possible uncontrolled variables. Careful planning is required for quasi-experimental designs, particularly in the identification of variables that may confound the demonstration of causal relationships. More details regarding these designs are given in Cook and Campbell (1979) and other references listed at the end of the chapter.

QUALITATIVE METHODS

Some gaps in knowledge concerning HCDs may require more information than is provided by the research designs previously described. Numerical information from standard group designs, quantitative descriptions, single-subject designs, and quasi-experimental designs may be too artificial and restricted. Information from observational and case study designs may be too superficial. In such cases, research methods borrowed from anthropology, sociology, and phenomenological psychology may be appropriate. These methods are described by terms such as *qualitative, ethnographic, sociolinguistic,* or *phenomenological.* Qualitative methods differ from group designs in several ways. They involve subjective qualitative rather than objective quantitative analyses, they often involve the study of individuals in natural settings, and the exact methods are not preplanned.

Qualitative research is not planned ahead in the manner of other research designs. Observations are made in a natural setting and carefully recorded. Observers attempt to suspend their own ideas and describe the situation from a number of different perspectives, including the point of view of the person or persons observed. The quality or "thickness" of the description comes from the use of multiple sources of information. In addition to observations, there may be interviews, diaries, and other types of information. As the researchers discover categories, subcategories, and components of meaning in the observations, broad 'themes" are expected to emerge that describe the major outlines of the phenomena observed. The findings could lead to the identification of independent and dependent variables for further study by quantitative research designs.

There are a variety of qualitative methods, and their procedures are difficult to describe in a concise manner. The methods have only recently been adopted by HCD researchers (cf. Pickering, 1984). Although qualitative methods may not be appropriate for obtaining information about all speech and hearing processes, there are important practical questions about HCDs that could be answered by gaining a deeper understanding of the communicative context of HCDs.

CONCLUSIONS REGARDING RESEARCH DESIGNS

In this book, like other books on research, it has been necessary to devote a great deal of space to the discussion of research designs. Only the most important characteristics of the most common designs have been given. Readers are directed to other sources for detailed information about research designs.

Research designs are often modified and combined to meet the needs of HCD research, as discussed in Chapter 17. The other research events are just as essential as the research design, but (with the exception of data analysis) they do not involve as much specialized technical information. There can be no research design without a problem and a specific purpose. Once the research has been designed, its contribution to knowledge depends on the efficacy of the procedure, the data analysis, and the interpretation, which are described next.

ADDITIONAL INFORMATION

All of the other designs, except qualitative methods, have been described by Shaughnessy and Zechmeister (1985). Further information about observational methods can be found in Hartmann (1982), Cochran, Moses, and Mosteller (1983), and Crano and Brewer (1986); case studies in Bromley (1986); descriptive methods in Fowler (1984); single-subject designs in Barlow, Hayes, and Nelson (1984), Barlow and Herson (1984), and Tawney and Gast (1984); single-subject designs in HCD research in Connell and Thompson (1986), Kearns (1986), and McReynolds and Thompson (1986), as well as McReynolds and Kearns (1983); quasi-experimental designs in Cook and Campbell (1979), Kratochwill (1978), and Cherulnik (1983); and qualitative methods in Spradley (1979), Polkinghorne (1983), Goetz and LeCompte (1984), Lofland and Lofland (1984), Taylor and Bogdan (1984), Giorgi (1985), and Howard (1985).

REVIEW QUESTIONS

1. List and briefly describe each of the other research designs discussed in this chapter.
2. Using the advantages and disadvantages of group designs discussed in Chapter 7 as a basis, discuss the advantages and disadvantages of observational methods, case study methods, single-subject designs, quasi-experimental designs, and qualitative methods.

CHAPTER

9

Procedures

After research is designed, further decisions must be made about the conditions of the study. These research events are described as the *procedure*. They involve exact definitions of the subject, situation, task, and treatment variables. The procedures are just as important as the design. The research contributes useful information only to the extent that the subjects, situations, tasks, and treatments are appropriate for the problem under investigation.

SUBJECTS

The design designates the kinds of subjects to be studied. The exact operations for selecting subjects are specified by the procedure. The subjects should be as representative as possible of those identified by the problem. Subject selection is limited by the availability of populations, and the availability of methods for determining relevant characteristics of the populations. The variables that dictate subject selection can be independent variables for comparing natural groups, control variables to be held constant within groups, or variables used to match groups. To meet these requirements of the design, subjects are selected according to predetermined criteria called *selection criteria*.

Selection criteria

Selection criteria can include age, sex, education, cultural background, history of treatment, abilities relevant to HCDs, presence or absence of HCDs, and types of HCDs. Age and sex can be specified without difficulty. Education, cultural background, and history of treatment are easily specified in general terms, but more precise definitions needed for certain studies may be difficult to formulate. Abilities relevant to HCDs may also be difficult to specify. For example, language abilities may have to be defined in terms of tests based on a particular theory of language.

Information concerning age, amount and type of education, history of treatment, and cultural background can be obtained from clinic records, school records, and interviews. Greater care is needed to determine educational achievement and abilities relevant to HCDs. Such information may be obtained from practitioners, teachers, and parents, from standardized tests, or by special assessment procedures devised by the researchers. Judgments of practitioners, teachers, and parents have ecological (external) validity, but may be unreliable. Standardized tests and special assessment procedures can provide more reliable information, but may be relatively crude and lack external validity.

The presence and the type of HCDs can be easily determined for some disorders. The hearing loss involved in conductive and sensorineural losses can usually be assessed by standard audiological tests in children and adults, and by special behavioral and physiological tests in infants. Speech disorders can be assessed by perceptual judgments of clinicians, by standard speech tests, or by acoustical analysis of speech.

Central auditory disorders and language disorders are not as easily defined, because they involve more central processes for which theoretical explanations are still being evolved. Acquired central auditory disorders are defined by evidence of brain dysfunction or by tests that are not yet well standardized. Developmental central auditory disorders are defined by the judgments of teachers and clinicians, and by tests that have not yet been well standardized. Acquired language disorders are defined by evidence of brain dysfunction, clinicians' judgments, standard tests, and special tests. Developmental language disorders are defined by the judgments of teachers and clinicians, standard tests, and special tests.

Obtaining Subjects

After selection criteria have been decided upon, it is necessary to determine whether the required numbers and types of subjects can be found. Where a certain type of HCD is to be studied, there may not be enough subjects in the most accessible clinics or schools. The researchers may have to obtain subjects from other clinics and schools, sometimes in very distant locations. In such cases, it is more difficult to control the conditions for testing and training. Alternatives are to collect data over a longer period of time, waiting until enough subjects become available in accessible locations to meet the requirements of the design, or to select a different design.

Studies of individuals may pose fewer problems of subject selection. However, researchers looking for rare cases, such as children with extreme language deprivation, would have to wait until enough cases had been found to complete the study. In surveys, special methods are used to select samples in order to ensure that the samples have representative distributions of relevant characteristics.

Sometimes the desired numbers and types of subjects cannot be obtained. Unless the study is abandoned or postponed, the design has to be modified. The number of independent variables can be reduced, the composition of groups altered, or the number of subjects per group decreased. This restricts the scope of the research and reduces the information obtained about the problem. In some cases, a *preliminary study* or *pilot study* that does not meet all of the requirements of the original design may be carried out.

Researchers must take a great deal of care to select the subjects specified by the design and the problem. This is not easy, but the success of the research depends on how well it is accomplished. Difficulties in meeting the subject requirements of research designs are almost unavoidable. Obtaining useful information with available subjects is one of the most challenging aspects of HCD research.

INDEPENDENT VARIABLES

The research design identifies the independent variables to be investigated. To put the design into operation, these variables must be precisely defined. Variables used as criteria for selecting subjects in some studies may serve as independent variables in others. Such variables would include age, sex, education, cultural background, history of treatment, abilities relevant to HCDs, presence or absence of HCDs, and types of HCDs. Just as in subject selection, some of these variables can be defined in a straightforward manner, and others are less easily defined. Great care must be taken in selecting procedures for defining independent variables of this type, to ensure that the levels of the independent variable have as much internal and external validity as possible.

The exact definition of independent variables involves special procedures devised by researchers to a greater extent than the definition of subject selection variables. The procedures may vary considerably as a function of the type of independent variables investigated. Some examples will be given here.

Hearing Variables

Hearing variables can be defined by standard audiological tests or by special procedures. These procedures can vary the acoustic and linguistic characteristics of sounds, and the acoustic and linguistic context in which the sounds are presented. Pure tones or complex sounds of different frequencies, intensities, and durations can be presented in quiet or in noise. Speech sounds, words, or connected speech can be filtered, compressed, or otherwise altered, presented to one or both ears in quiet, or with competing noise or speech.

The listening task can require the subject to detect, discriminate, or integrate the sounds that are presented. This can be accomplished by the use of physiological, psychophysical, or psychometric testing procedures. Operant conditioning procedures can be used to test the hearing of infants. Almost all of these tasks are presented in conditions where background sounds are carefully controlled. Only rarely are hearing variables assessed in natural situations.

Psychoacoustic procedures for assessing detection and discrimination are well established, as are operant conditioning procedures and some physiological procedures such as impedance audiometry. Other physiological procedures such as evoked response audiometry are not yet well established. Nor are psychometric procedures for assessing central auditory processes involved in integration and perception. The goal of research may be to develop reliable and valid testing procedures, in order that such procedures can be used in later research on the characteristics of disorders.

In research on hearing disorders, the usefulness of the findings will depend on the validity of the measures of hearing. There is less difficulty in assessing peripheral aspects of hearing, but more adequate theories of central auditory processes are needed to serve as a basis for the development of valid central auditory tests.

Language Variables

Language variables may be defined for language reception, language expression, and communicative interactions. Special procedures may be needed to define a particular level of language such as the phonetic, phonological, lexical, syntactic, semantic, discourse, or pragmatic level.

Receptive or expressive language variables can be particular language levels (e.g., speech sounds, nonsense words, words, or sentences) in carefully controlled communicative contexts or in more natural communicative settings.

Receptive language tasks can require subjects to discriminate, identify, comprehend, or repeat the linguistic stimuli that are presented at particular language levels, or receptive abilities can be assessed on the basis of interactive responses during communication. Expressive language tasks can require subjects to repeat linguistic stimuli at particular levels, describe pictures, describe past events in their lives, respond to questions, retell stories, or engage in more natural communicative interactions.

A number of standard aphasia tests for acquired language disorders and standard language tests for developmental disorders are available, and new tests are devised on the basis of new language theories. These tests are not as well established as tests of peripheral hearing, but have a firmer theoretical basis than central auditory tests. Special procedures for assessing language abilities have been devised by linguists and psycholinguists as well as by HCD researchers. Neurolinguists devise procedures for relating language and brain functioning.

The exact procedures used for assessing language are of great importance for interpreting research on language disorders. The problem, the research design, and the exact procedures used to evaluate language interact to determine the kind of information about language disorders that can be contributed by research. The value of the information depends on the ingenuity of researchers in developing special procedures, as well as the research design selected, and the nature of the problem.

Speech Variables

Acoustic, linguistic, physiological, or motor characteristics of speech variables may be defined for research on speech disorders. The speech can be speech sounds, syllables, words, sentences, or connected speech in controlled or natural settings.

Speaking tasks can require subjects to repeat, name pictures, answer questions, tell stories, or engage in more natural communicative activities. Well-established procedures are available for assessing articulation, stuttering, voice disorders, and cleft palate. Special procedures have been developed for assessing specific aspects of these disorders, such as movements of the vocal musculature, physiological activity during speech, changes in the vocal cavities, acoustic characteristics of speech, and the effects of communicative demands on speech.

In research on speech disorders there is less problem regarding the validity of procedures, as speech variables can be assessed more directly than hearing and language variables. However, speech involves complex movements and changes in the vocal cavity, as well as complex relationships to language variables, and the speech theories on which research procedures are based continue to evolve.

Treatment Variables

Independent variables in HCD research also include treatment variables. The operations used for treatments and for control conditions involving no treatment or alternative treatments must be specified. These operations include the exact type of treatment, the frequency and duration of treatment, and the criteria for terminating treatment.

Treatments might involve communication aids such as hearing aids, or training procedures such as repetition of speech sounds, naming, answering questions, and more natural communicative activities. The success of treatment can be evaluated by comparisons with control groups, changes in target behaviors after treatment, *generalization* to nontarget behaviors, *carry-over* to natural communication situations, and *maintenance* of treatment effects. Treatments may involve standard clinical methods or special methods developed by researchers.

The evaluation of treatments is a very important type of HCD research. The external validity of treatment methods, that is, the extent to which they improve communication in natural settings, is particularly important.

Other Independent Variables

Other independent variables in HCD research relate to the consequences of HCDs, as opposed to their primary defining characteristics. These include procedures for self-evaluating HCDs, and procedures for assessing the effects of HCDs on personal adjustment and on educational and vocational achievement. Research involving such variables is becoming much more common.

DEPENDENT VARIABLES

Exact procedures must be specified for defining the dependent variables that indicate the effects of independent variables. Dependent variables indicative of hearing include physiological responses to sounds, and the detection, discrimination, and identification of sounds by spoken, written, or choice responses. Dependent variables indicative of language include spoken, written, or choice responses to test items, language samples obtained in various ways, and communicative interactions. Dependent variables indicative of speech include speech, movements of the vocal musculature, physiological responses, and breathing responses.

Reliability of Judgments of Dependent Variables

Where objective measures of dependent variables are recorded, there are usually no questions regarding the reliability of measurement. Where dependent variables are subjective judgments of observers, it may be necessary to demonstrate that different observers make similar judgments. This can be done by having two or more observers record their judgments of an on-going experimental situation, audiotaped or videotaped responses, acoustic representations of speech, or other forms of spoken response. The degree to which observers agree is called *interobserver reliability* and is usually calculated in terms of the percentage of agreement between observers. In some cases, extensive training of judges is necessary to achieve acceptable reliability.

TASKS

The experimental tasks may be standard procedures for determining hearing, language, and speech abilities, or special tasks may be used. The task may be an important determinant of the information needed for the research. If one particular ability is to be assessed without involving other abilities, special care may be needed in selecting or devising tasks. For example, to test vocabulary without requiring spoken definitions from speech impaired subjects, a multiple choice task may be used where the subject points to a picture in response to a spoken word.

EQUIPMENT

Some studies require a great deal of equipment and others, very little. This can be an important practical consideration for procedure. For some research, the main focus may be on designing, obtaining, and assessing equipment. Researchers may have to obtain funds for expensive equipment, appropriate space for housing bulky equipment, and technical assistance for constructing, operating, and maintaining complex equipment. Equipment may be used to present tasks, record responses, and analyze findings.

Equipment Used for Task Presentation

Equipment used to present tasks can be clinic equipment such as diagnostic and training devices used for hearing tests, speech and language diagnosis and therapy, and education of children who are hearing impaired. Special-purpose equipment designed by researchers may also be used. Visual stimuli may be presented with printed tests, picture cards, slides, videotapes, or computer displays. Auditory stimuli can be presented through earphones or loudspeakers from audiometers, audiotapes, electronic tone generators, speech synthesizers, or computers. Considerable time and expertise may be necessary to prepare and record stimuli. Special calibration procedures may be necessary to ensure that sounds are presented at the desired frequency, intensity, and duration.

Equipment Used for Recording Responses

Spoken responses and communicative interactions can be recorded by audiotape or videotape. Choice responses are recorded by electrical, electronic, or computer devices. Physiological responses are recorded by electrophysiological devices specially designed for hearing, language, and speech responses. Speech movements and breathing are recorded by special electronic and electromechanical devices.

Equipment Used for Data Analysis

Equipment may be needed for various forms of data analysis. Spoken responses may be reproduced as visual representations of acoustic wave forms. The accuracy and speed of choice responses may be directly computed. Certain characteristics of language samples may be automatically analyzed. Numerical averages of physiological responses to repetitive stimuli may be calculated. Statistical analyses of numerical data may be carried out. Such data analyses may greatly improve the sensitivity of data analyses and save researchers a great deal of time.

The Role of Computers

Computers began to play a role in research when laboratory computers became available about 20 years ago. Few researchers could obtain these bulky and expensive instruments. With advances in computer technology, relatively inexpensive microcomputers are now available that can perform the functions of laboratory computers. Microcomputer systems are being developed for synthesizing and presenting stimuli, and for recording and analyzing data. Of particular interest are computer programs for synthesizing and analyzing speech, analyzing language samples, recognizing speech, and augmenting communication. Such computer applications will expand and facilitate HCD research.

SITUATIONS FOR OBSERVATION, TESTING, AND TRAINING

The situation in which the research is carried out is an important aspect of procedure. Quiet, distraction-free testing and training conditions necessary for some research may be difficult to arrange in schools and clinics. Special testing rooms may be needed for auditory and physiological research.

Research procedures may involve a specific set of operations carried out by specially trained personnel. Exact instructions and exact sequences of test operations may be essential to the purposes of research. *Double-blind* procedures may be needed to ensure that neither the researchers nor the subjects are aware which levels of the independent variable are being presented. Special procedures may be needed to minimize practice effects, fatigue, and boredom. In general, the researchers or research assistants who carry out the research must be well trained, punctual, and consistent, must understand the processes that are being studied, and must carry out operations exactly as prescribed.

In observational studies, special care may be needed to ensure that the situation is as natural as possible, and that the observer or recording system intrudes as little as possible.

LIMITATIONS IMPOSED BY PROCEDURES

Knowledge obtained by research is limited not only by designs, as discussed in Chapters 7 and 8, but by procedures. The findings must be interpreted with regard to the exact subject, situation, task, and treatment variables that have been defined by decisions about procedures. Researchers should be as aware of the limitations on knowledge imposed by procedures as they are of the limitations imposed by designs.

ADDITIONAL INFORMATION

Information about specific procedures can be found in published research on the topic in question, where further references regarding the source of procedures may be given.

REVIEW QUESTION

1. In the research reports in a recent issue of *JSHR* or *JSHD*, find the exact specifications for subjects, independent variables, dependent variables, tasks, equipment, and situations. Note any limitations imposed by these procedures on the knowledge that was obtained.

CHAPTER
10

Data Reduction and Descriptive Statistics

Af, fter the procedures have been carried out, the researchers have collected the basic information or *raw data*. The raw data are the measures or observations of the dependent variable, which could be spoken, signed, written, choice, movement, or physiological responses. There is almost always some analysis of data prior to interpretation. The first phase of data analysis is usually *data reduction*, where the aspects of the dependent variables that will be analyzed are expressed in the form required for analysis. Where the data have been expressed in numerical form, the next phase of analysis may be to organize or summarize them to obtain *descriptive statistics* that provide useful information about the characteristics of the data.

DATA REDUCTION

Some types of data reduction are simple and rapid. Others are difficult and time-consuming, and may require expensive and elaborate equipment. Where subjective judgments are involved, estimates of the reliability of the judgments may be required. Data reduction should be taken into consideration in planning research, because researchers may not have the time or facilities necessary for data reduction.

Spoken or Signed Responses: Written Transcriptions

Where the raw data are spoken or signed responses, the first step may be to *transcribe* the responses into written form as words, syllables, or phonetic symbols. This can be one of the most time-consuming aspects of the research. Special procedures may be needed to ensure the reliability of the transcriptions.

The next stage of data reduction for transcribed responses depends on the purpose of the research. The written transcripts may be classified according to their phonetic, phonological, lexical, syntactic, semantic, pragmatic, or other characteristics. These classification procedures may be simple and rapid, or complex and time-consuming. Simple classifications might involve only the determination of correctness of a repetition response, or the correctness of spoken responses to items on standard hearing, language, or speech tests. More complex classifications could be estimation of vocabulary size, determination of the relative frequency of use of grammatical classes, and assessment of discourse and pragmatic skills. Where classifications require subjective judgments, procedures for assessing the reliability of judgments may be needed.

Classifications of spoken responses are often numerical representations of the dependent variable, such as percent correct phonemes or words, or frequency of use of different grammatical classes, discourse devices, or pragmatic strategies. These numerical quantities can be used for descriptive statistics, as will be described. Where further analyses are not quantitative, there is some form of qualitative analysis, as described in Chapter 15.

Spoken Responses: Acoustic Representations

Acoustic representations of spoken responses may be recorded as *spectrograms*, which show changes in sound spectra during speech. The phonetic and phonological characteristics and the quality of vocalizations may be judged subjectively by direct observations that require reliability estimates. Sophisticated computer analyses may also be used to obtain objective quantitative estimates of vocal characteristics such as hoarseness and linguistic characteristics such as formant structure. The computer analyses enable researchers to reduce data rapidly and obtain precise objective information.

Written Responses

Written responses can be classified in the same way as spoken responses with regard to correctness, frequency of usage, and assessment of skills. For certain purposes, the quality of the handwriting may also be assessed. Where subjective judgments of written responses are involved, reliability estimates may be required.

Choice Responses

Data reduction is simpler for choice responses. The response can be a spoken, written, or button-pushing response to indicate detection, discrimination, or identification of stimuli such as pure tones, speech, pictures, or tactile vibrations. Where the responses are spoken or written, they are classified by the listener or reader as correct or incorrect. The speed and accuracy of button-pushing responses can be recorded automatically, thus saving a great deal of time and effort.

Movements

Movements of the speech musculature and other movements can be directly observed, with data reduction through subjective judgments. However, movements are often recorded by sensing devices and either displayed on graphs or in numerical form that can be used for descriptive statistics.

Physiological Responses

Physiological responses may be recorded as changes in mechanical or electrical activity that are displayed on screens or printed out to permit researchers to make subjective judgments of dependent variables such as brainstem responses to pure tones. Data reduction may be part of the recording procedure, as is the case for the averaging of brainstem responses to a series of pure tones. Descriptive statistics may be based on subjective judgments of visual representations of physiological responses, or on numerical data.

DESCRIPTIVE STATISTICS

Descriptive statistics organize and summarize data. They are useful for the interpretation of statistical analyses, and may be the final form of data analysis in studies that do not require statistical analysis. Organization may involve ranking, frequency distributions, and tabular or graphic displays. Summaries involve measures of central tendency and variability.

Ranking

Numerical data can be organized into a more useful form by ranking. Ranked scores are easier to assess than unranked scores, as shown in Table 10–1.

Frequency Distributions

Where there is a large amount of ranked data, more useful information is provided by grouping the ranked data into *frequency distributions*, as shown in Table 10–2. Frequency distributions can provide a great deal of information. In Table 10–2, it can easily be seen that the HCD subjects tend to have lower scores clustered in the range 0–19 and the non-HCD subjects have higher scores in the range 10–29. It is also important to be aware of the overlap between groups. Some HCD subjects score as high or higher than non-HCD subjects. When only measures of central tendency are presented, they may be misinterpreted as indicating that all members of one group are superior to all members of another group.

Frequency distributions also provide important information about the *shape* of the data. The distributions in Table 10–2 are fairly *normal*. The scores cluster around a midpoint and become less frequent on either side. Frequency distributions may also be nonnormal or *skewed*. The most common forms of skewed distributions in HCD research occur when the majority of scores cluster at the high or the low end of the frequency distribution. Distributions with a large proportion of near-maximum scores are said to have *ceiling effects* and those with a large proportion of near-minimum scores are said to have *floor effects*, as shown in Table 10–3. It is essential to be aware of ceiling and floor effects. They decrease the possibility of demonstrating the effects of independent variables, because scores are limited by the ceiling or the floor. Less powerful statistical tests must be

TABLE 10–1.
Ranking of Numerical Data.

Unranked	Ranked
23	4
4	8
13	13
8	23

TABLE 10–2.
Frequency Distributions of Ranked Data.

Scores	Frequency of Scores	
	HCD	Non-HCD
0–4	8	0
5–9	11	3
10–14	16	7
15–19	9	13
20–24	2	15
25–29	0	7
30–34	0	1

used for comparing skewed distributions, and the correlations between variables cannot be adequately assessed where there are skewed distributions.

Central Tendency and Variability

The main trends of numerical data can be summarized by measures of *central tendency* and measures of *variability*. Measures of central tendency include *means* or averages, *medians* or middle ranks, and *modes* or most frequent numbers. Measures of variability include the *range* of the ranked measures and the *standard deviation* of the measures. Each of these measures is illustrated in Table 10–4. Because the numbers are distributed in a fairly normal manner, the measures of central tendency are about the same. The average can be rounded off to 6, the middlemost ranked number is 6, and the most frequent or modal number is 6. The two measures of variability assess different aspects of the distribution. The range indicates the complete extent of the distribution by listing the lowest and the highest number. The standard deviation estimates how much the

TABLE 10–3.
Skewed Frequency Distributions.

		Ceiling Effect	Floor Effect
Minimum	0–19	0	26
	20–39	3	14
	40–59	7	9
	60–79	18	1
Maximum	80–99	22	0

TABLE 10–4.
Measures of Central Tendency and Variability.

Scores		
1		Mean (average) = 5.7
3		Median (middlemost ranked number) = 6
3	Central Tendency:	Mode (most frequent number) = 6
5		
6		
6		
6	Variability:	Range = 1 to 10
8		Standard Deviation = 2.82
9		
10		

scores vary from the mean. A standard deviation of 2.82 estimates that 68 percent of the numbers would fall in a region 2.82 above and 2.82 below the mean. This region includes the numbers 3 to 8. Since 7 (70 percent) of the 10 numbers fall in this region, the standard deviation is an accurate estimate of variability even in small samples, providing the data are distributed in a fairly normal manner.

It is always useful to look at frequency distributions, as measures of central tendency and variability do not directly indicate the presence of ceiling and floor effects.

Transformations

Some numerical data are systematically skewed in such a way that measures of central tendency and variability are misleading, and the most powerful statistical tests cannot be used. It may be possible to *transform* the scores in such a way that the skewed distribution becomes more normal. For example, where reaction times are the dependent variable, the distribution usually clusters around a minimum reaction time and there is a wide dispersion of long reaction times. The distribution can be made more normal by transforming the reaction times to reciprocals, logarithms, or square roots.

Tables and Graphs

Rankings, frequency distributions, and measures of central tendency and reliability can be presented in the form of tables and graphs for easier inspection of trends. For questionnaires and surveys, the presentation of raw data and descriptive statistics is often the final stage of data analysis.

A great deal of care must be taken in the preparation of tables and graphs to make the information readily available to those who wish to use it.

ADDITIONAL INFORMATION

Data reduction takes many different forms, depending on the type of research. The most useful information may often be found in published research reports. Published reports may also give references for further information regarding specific techniques of data reduction. General discussions of data reduction and descriptive statistics can be found in books on research methods, research design, and statistics. Readers are particularly directed to Fallik and Brown (1983) and Tufte (1983).

REVIEW QUESTIONS

1. Why must the requirements for data reduction be considered when planning research?
2. List the kinds of data reduction that may be involved in HCD research.
3. Identify the types of data reduction that were used in the research reports in a recent issue of *JSHR* or *JSHD*.
4. List the kinds of descriptive statistics that are used in HCD research.
5. What information is given by frequency distributions that is not given by measures of central tendency?
6. Why is it important to be aware of floor effects and ceiling effects?
7. Find the descriptive statistics in the research reports in a recent issue of *JSHR* or *JSHD*.

CHAPTER
11

Basic Principles of Statistical Analysis

S tatistical analyses of research data estimate the probability that the observed effects of varying the independent variable could have occurred by chance. These probability estimates provide a means of deciding how confidently the research findings can be accepted as knowledge regarding HCDs. Where relationships between variables are studied, statistical analyses also indicate how closely the variables are related. Information about relationships is more difficult to interpret with regard to new knowledge about HCDs. The basic principles of statistical analysis will be described in this chapter, the statistical analysis of simple group designs will be described in the next chapter, and then the statistical analysis of complex group designs, the statistical analysis of relationships, and the methods of analyses used for other designs will be described in the following chapters.

Formal coursework in statistics is usually essential for those who wish to carry out HCD research, and also for those who wish to evaluate research with regard to practical applications. Even when statistics courses have been completed, it is often difficult to apply the techniques that have been learned to HCD research. An overview of the applications of statistical analyses in HCD research is given in this and the following chapters. Further insight into this important but difficult aspect of research can be gained by reading published research and consulting statisticians who are familiar with HCD research problems.

PLANNING STATISTICAL ANALYSES

As far as possible, the statistical analyses should be planned at the time the study is designed. The probability estimates that indicate the degree of confidence in the knowledge resulting from research are only valid when decisions about data analysis are made before the data are gathered. When decisions are made after the data have been examined, researchers may consciously or unconsciously organize or select data that show the desired effects. Such biased data analyses provide false knowledge that could mislead practitioners and persons with HCDs.

There are exceptions to the requirement for preplanning statistical analyses. In many studies it is not possible to predict the shape of the distributions of data. Where distributions are badly skewed, alternative forms of statistical analysis may be required; where relationships among variables are complex, additional methods of analysis may be needed to estimate the interrelationships of the variables. Such changes in statistical planning should not introduce bias in the form of reorganization or selection. Researchers must always guard against bias in statistical analyses in the same manner that they take special precautions to ensure the reliability of observations and subjective judgments. When statistical analyses are properly planned, the research findings will have maximum practical benefits.

SELECTION OF STATISTICAL TECHNIQUES

Another reason why planning is necessary is that the statistical techniques must be appropriate to the design, procedure, and data reduction requirements. As much as possible, decisions about these research events should be made at the same time. If an appropriate statistical technique is not available for a particular set of design, procedure, and data reduction requirements, it may be necessary to modify the study to fit available statistical techniques. Researchers who are not familiar with the full range of statistical techniques will be limited in their ability to plan research that contributes the most useful information. In the absence of such knowledge, statistical techniques can be selected by consulting a statistician, but the global planning that takes all events into consideration at the same time may not be possible.

STATISTICAL POWER

An important consideration in selecting statistical tests is to select the most *powerful* test possible. Powerful tests are those that are most sensitive to the effects of varying the independent variable. In formal mathematical terms, statistical tests are tests of the *null hypothesis* that there is no effect of varying the independent variable. Powerful, sensitive tests are those that most often reject the null hypothesis when there is an effect. Where data are distributed adequately, powerful statistical tests called *parametric tests* can be used. Where data are not distributed adequately, it may be necessary to use less powerful tests called *nonparametric tests*. The more familiar researchers are with considerations of statistical power, the more effective will be their research planning.

STATISTICAL SIGNIFICANCE

The outcome of a statistical test is a statement of the probability that the observed effect of the independent variable could have occurred by chance. In Table 11–1, the independent variable is the occurrence or non-occurrence of an HCD in independent groups, and the dependent variable is the score on a language test. The HCD mean of 13.5 is lower than the non-HCD mean of 19.0, but the groups are small and the distributions overlap. A statistical test of the observed effect will result in a statement of the probability that the difference between means could have occurred by chance. In planning the statistical analysis, the researchers should decide on the level of chance occurrence that they will accept. In almost all HCD

TABLE 11–1.
Hypothetical Scores on a Language Test.

HCD Group	Non-HCD Group
8	10
9	14
11	18
16	25
23	28

research, this level of chance, called the *level of confidence* or the *level of statistical significance* is set at a probability of .05 or .01. The .05 level indicates that only 5 times in 100 would the observed difference between means occur by chance. The .01 level sets the chance level at 1 time in 100.

Since the object of HCD research is to contribute useful knowledge about HCDs, the statistical significance of the findings is crucial. Researchers attempt to design experiments, devise procedures, and select methods of data analysis that will lead to significant differences. The choice of the level of confidence is determined by practical considerations. In the earlier stages of research on a problem, the more liberal .05 or 5 percent level may be selected to guide further research. In the later stages of research, and particularly when there are large groups of subjects, the more conservative .01 level may be selected in order that new knowledge may be accepted with greater confidence. Once the level of confidence has been selected, it cannot be changed. A probability of .053 that "approaches" the .05 level is *not* statistically significant. Similarly, if the .05 level of significance has been chosen, it cannot be said that a difference is significant at a different level, that is, "significant at the .10 level."

ACCEPTING OR REJECTING THE NULL HYPOTHESIS

When an observed difference between means is found to be statistically significant at the preselected level of confidence, the researchers can reject the null hypothesis, which states that there is no effect of the independent variable. However, when the difference between means is not significant, they cannot *accept* the null hypothesis and conclude that there is no effect of the independent variable. A nonsignificant effect could occur even when there actually is an effect. For example, the measures obtained from a language test may be too crude to demonstrate the effects of language training in a comparison of a trained and nontrained group. Similarly, skewed distributions of scores might reduce the observed effects, resulting in a misleadingly small difference in means.

It is important to be aware of the potential dangers of accepting the null hypothesis. Accepting the null hypothesis is probably the most common error in HCD research. There are practical reasons for wanting to accept the null hypothesis. It is very useful to show that a more rapid training procedure produces the same benefits as a slower procedure, or that HCD groups do not differ from non-HCD groups in certain skills. However, this knowledge cannot be obtained by interpreting nonsignificant differences as proving that no difference exists. More complicated research strategies are needed to demonstrate similarities, as indicated in Chapter 17.

There is an equal danger in accepting the null hypothesis with regard to nonsignificant relationships in correlation designs. Correlational measures of relationships are evaluated according to their statistical significance, but nonsignificant relationships should not be interpreted as a complete lack of relationship. If a nonsignificant correlation is found between hearing loss and amount of noise exposure, it should not be concluded that noise exposure is not dangerous. The measure of noise exposure or the measure of hearing loss may have been too crude to indicate a subtle relationship, correlated variables may have confounded the relationship, or variability may have been limited by ceiling or floor effects.

This seemingly technical point regarding the null hypothesis is of crucial importance for the practical application of knowledge obtained from research. The null hypothesis provides another example of why all research events should be considered in planning research. If the stated purpose of research is to demonstrate no difference between groups or no relationship between variables, the researchers must be aware that this purpose cannot be accomplished by simply obtaining a nonsignificant result on a statistical test.

NUMBER OF SUBJECTS REQUIRED FOR STATISTICAL ANALYSES

As stated in relation to research design, it is important to select enough subjects to meet the requirements for statistical analyses. The minimum requirements vary from a desirable minimum of 10 subjects per cell to an absolute minimum of 5 subjects per cell of the design. A 2×3 design would have 6 cells and require a minimum of 30 to 60 subjects. A $2 \times 3 \times 4$ design would have 24 cells and require a minimum of 120 to 240 subjects. It is easy to see why the kinds of complex designs that are suitable to the complexity of problems concerning HCDs are difficult to put into operation. It is important to consider the statistical requirements at the time of designing the research. Researchers should make every effort to carry out preliminary research that will indicate which variables should be focused on, and simplify designs to permit acceptable statistical analyses with available subjects.

ADDITIONAL INFORMATION

Most books on research design and statistics discuss the basic principles of statistical analysis (cf. Clayton, 1984; Fallik & Brown, 1983; Kirk, 1984; Spence, Cotton, Underwood, & Duncan, 1983).

REVIEW QUESTIONS

1. Give two reasons why it is important to plan statistical analyses at the time of designing the research.
2. Why must statistical power be considered in planning data analyses?
3. What is the null hypothesis?
4. What is statistical significance?
5. Why is the choice of the level of confidence important?
6. Why should researchers not accept the null hypothesis?
7. Why is it important to consider the number of subjects per cell when planning research?

CHAPTER
12

Statistical Analysis of Simple Group Designs

S tatistical analyses of simple group designs estimate the significance of the difference between the two levels of the independent variable. For independent group designs, the significance of the difference between groups is estimated, and for repeated measurement designs the significance of the differences between two conditions for one group is estimated. The choice of statistical test depends on the type of design and the form of the distribution of responses. If there is a significant difference, the null hypothesis is rejected and it is concluded that there is a probable effect of the independent variable at the preselected level (.05 or .01) of confidence. If there is not a significant difference, the null hypothesis is not rejected, and it is concluded that the effect of the independent variable has not been demonstrated.

INDEPENDENT GROUP DESIGNS

Relatively simple statistical tests are used to analyze the data collected with independent group designs, where the effect of an independent variable of groups is isolated by controlling relevant variables. These tests can be used with simple random selection, random assignment, matched group, and natural group designs.

A hypothetical study will illustrate the statistical procedures. The independent variable is age of beginning language instruction. A group of 10 children who are hearing impaired and began language instruction before the age of 2 is compared with a group of 10 children who are hearing impaired and began language instruction after the age of 5. All subjects are 8 years old at the time of testing. The dependent variable is a simple test of language ability, number of words used to describe a picture. The results for individual children in each group are shown in Table 12–1.

The first thing to note is that there is one score for each subject in each group. The statistical analysis of simple independent group designs is based on one score per subject, no more and no less. All of the information that can be obtained from a simple independent group design is derived from these two sets of scores. The statistical test could not be simply a comparison of group means, because the means do not reflect the variability of the distributions.

Inspection of the data indicates a larger number of words in the picture descriptions of the early instruction group, but a number of overlapping scores for the two groups. A statistical test is needed to determine the probability that the difference between the two distributions of scores could have occurred by chance. The most powerful statistical tests estimate the probability by comparing the difference between means to the variability of scores within each group. This procedure is the most powerful because it makes use of all the data.

It is easy to see how these statistical tests work. If all the children in the early group had received scores of 24 or 25 and all the children in the late group had received scores of 18 or 19, the mean difference would be the same but the variability within groups would be much smaller and the probability of a chance difference would be much smaller. If the scores had ranged from 0 to 50 in the early group and from 0 to 40 in the second group with the same group means, the variability within groups would have been greater and the probability of a chance difference would have been larger. The relationship between differences in central tendency and variability within groups is more easily seen when the distributions are plotted as in Table 12–2.

The t-Test for Independent Measures

A statistical test is necessary to estimate the probability that the difference between distributions could have occurred by chance. The most powerful test for differences between two independent groups is a *parametric test*, the *t-test for independent measures*. The calculations are

TABLE 12–1.
Hypothetical Results on a Language Test for two Independent Groups.

	Early Instruction	Later Instruction
	34	27
	31	25
	30	23
	28	20
	26	18
	24	17
	22	16
	19	15
	18	13
	16	11
MEAN	24.8	18.5

very simple, and can be done with a pocket calculator or a computer program. The difference between means (24.8 minus 18.5, or 6.30) is divided by a number based on the within-group variance (2.52). The resulting t ratio is 2.50 (6.30/2.52), indicating that the measure of the effect of the independent variable was 2.50 times as large as the measure of the variability of the groups. Reference to a table of t ratios reveals that the probability of such a difference occurring by chance is less than .05 for two groups of 10 subjects. The difference between groups would be statistically significant if the .05 level of confidence had been selected by researchers, but not if the .01 level had been selected. If the difference between groups had been larger or the variability within groups smaller, the t ratio would have been larger and the probability of chance differences smaller.

This simple example provides a good illustration of the importance of planning all aspects of research at the same time. The choice of the level of significance is important. If this were one of a number of studies on the same topic, the .01 level of confidence would have been chosen and the difference between groups would not have been significant. To increase the chances of a significant difference, the variability within groups might have been reduced by more rigorous criteria for selecting subjects, and the difference between means might have been increased by the use of a more sensitive test of language ability. To interpret a significant difference as the effect of the independent variable, a natural groups variable, it must, of course, be assumed that all other relevant variables had been adequately controlled.

TABLE 12-2.
Distribution of Language Test Scores from Table 12-1.

Number of Words	Early Instruction	Later Instruction
34	x	
33		
32		
31	x	
30	x	
29		
28	x	
27		x
26	x	
25	MEAN	x
24	x	
23		x
22	x	
21		
20		x
19	x	MEAN
18	x	x
17		x
16	x	x
15		x
14		
13		x
12		
11		x

This example also illustrates the danger of accepting the null hypothesis. If the .01 level were used, the null hypothesis would not be rejected. It should not be concluded that early language training has no effect on language acquisition, but that the effect was not proven. In the hypothetical study, it is almost certain that such an effect would be demonstrated if subjects were adequately matched and the measure of language ability was sufficiently sensitive.

Partitioning Variances

In the descriptions of analysis of variance in the next two chapters, statistical analyses will be discussed in terms of *partitioning* of variances. The same terminology can be applied to the *t*-test to illustrate the similarity between the statistical analyses of simple and complex group designs. For the data in Table 12–1, *total* variance would be calculated for the 20 measures in the combined groups. Then the total variance would be *partitioned* into two components—the *between* variance (difference between the means of the two groups) and the *within* variance (variance of scores within each group). For both simple and group designs, the likelihood of statistically significant differences increases as *between* variance becomes larger or *within* variance becomes smaller and decreases as *between* variance becomes smaller or *within* variance larger.

One-Tailed Tests

To increase the power of the *t*-test, a *one-tailed test* might have been used. With this procedure, a prediction is made that the two means can differ in only one direction. In the present example, it might be predicted that if the groups differed at all in picture naming, the early instruction group would use more words. If this one-tailed prediction were made, the probability of a chance difference for a given *t* ratio would be reduced by half. In the present example, the probability of chance difference would have been reduced from .05 to .025.

The one-tailed test is a procedure that appeals to researchers who wish to increase statistical power. However, the predicted direction of difference must *always* be specified before the data are collected, and the researchers must be willing to ignore mean differences in the nonpredicted direction. In the early stages of research on a given problem, it is best to sacrifice statistical power and allow for mean differences in both directions. See the sections on *Planned Comparisons* in the next chapter for a further discussion of this research strategy.

Nonparametric Tests of Simple Independent Group Designs

Parametric statistical tests like the *t*-test are based on the assumption that the distributions of scores are normal and the variances (standard deviations squared) of the two distributions are equal. However, statisticians have found that with groups of equal size, the distributions can be markedly skewed and the variances quite different without affecting the validity of the test.

Even where liberal criteria for normal distributions and equal variances are used, it may be difficult to meet the criteria in HCD research. HCD groups tend to have more widely scattered scores than non-HCD groups. If the experimental task is too easy for the non-HCD group, their near-perfect scores can result in a ceiling effect, and if the task is too difficult for the HCD group, their low scores can result in a floor effect.

When the distributions of scores do not meet the requirements for parametric tests, *nonparametric tests* can be used. These tests do not assume normal distributions and equal variance. The less strict requirements involve a loss of statistical power. Nonparametric tests are less powerful than parametric tests, because they do not make use of all the information about variability to estimate the probability of differences between groups.

The most powerful nonparametric tests use data that have been transformed to ranks. A nonparametric rank test for two independent groups is the *Mann-Whitney* or *Sum of Ranks Test*. The scores for both groups are ranked together, and the probability of a difference between groups is based on a difference between the sum of the ranks for the two groups. In the previous example, the scores would be ranked as shown in Table 12–3. The sum of ranks reflects both the central tendency and the variability (i.e., the overlapping ranks) of the two distributions. When the simple calculations for the Mann-Whitney Test have been carried out, it can be determined that the difference between groups is significant at the .05 level, demonstrating that the Mann-Whitney Test was as powerful as the *t*-test for these particular data.

Nonparametric tests that use frequencies or categories are less powerful than rank tests. For two independent groups, a test based on frequencies is called the *Median Test*. The two groups are compared simply in terms of the number of scores falling above and not above the median for the combined groups. The combined group median in the previous example is 21 words. Seven scores in the early instruction group and three scores in the late instruction group fall above the median, and three scores in the early group and seven scores in the late group do not fall above the median, as shown in Table 12–4. The probability that such a difference could have

TABLE 12–3.
Language Test Results from Table 12–1 Transformed to Ranks.

	Early Instruction		Late Instruction	
	Words	Rank	Words	Rank
	34	20	27	16
	31	19	25	14
	30	18	23	12
	28	17	20	10
	26	15	18	7.5
	24	13	17	6
	22	11	16	4.5
	19	9	15	3
	18	7.5	13	2
	16	4.5	11	1
Sum of Ranks		134		76

TABLE 12–4.
Median Test Scores from Table 12–1.

	Early	Late
Above the Median	7	3
Not Above the Median	3	7

occurred by chance, as determined by a procedure called *Fisher's Exact Method*, is not significant at the .05 level. With exactly the same data, then, the difference between groups becomes nonsignificant when a less powerful test is used.

REPEATED MEASUREMENT DESIGNS

The *t*-Test for Correlated Measures

Statistical tests for simple repeated measurement designs are very similar to the tests for independent groups. The most common parametric test for repeated measurement of two levels of an independent variable is the *t-test for correlated measures*. The test is also called the *t-test for paired observations*, and can be used when there are matched pairs of subjects in two independent groups. The statistic is calculated by relating the difference between means to the variability of differences between the paired measures. The greater the number of differences that favor one condition, the larger will be the *t* ratio, and the greater the probability of a significant difference. In the example shown in Table 12–5, the difference between

TABLE 12–5.
Hypothetical Results of Two Tests for a Single Group.

Subject	Test 1	Test 2	Difference
1	95	90	5
2	86	93	−7
3	90	88	2
4	73	77	−4
5	65	74	−9
6	78	80	−2
7	86	95	−9
8	82	80	2
9	87	87	0
10	72	65	7
Mean	81.4	82.9	

correlated means would not be statistically significant ($t = 0.83$) because the measure of the variability among difference scores (1.81) is large relative to the difference between means (1.5).

Non-parametric Tests of Simple Repeated Measurement Designs

A nonparametric test for repeated measures that uses ranked data is the *Wilcoxen Signed Rank Test for Paired Observations*. The differences between the repeated measures or paired observations are ranked from smallest to largest without regard to the direction of the difference. Then the ranks for positive and negative differences are summed separately. Once again, the greater the number of differences that favor one condition, the more likely a significant difference. In many cases, this test is almost as powerful as the *t*-test.

The least powerful test for repeated measurements and paired observations is the *Sign test*. Only the direction of differences between measures is used, and the greater the number of differences that favor one condition, the greater the likelihood of a significant difference.

ADDITIONAL INFORMATION

Additional information about statistical tests used for simple group designs can be found in elementary statistics texts (cf. Clayton, 1984; Fallik & Brown, 1983; Kirk, 1984; Spence, Cotton, Underwood, & Duncan, 1983). Simple step-by-step procedures for statistical calculations with a pocket calculator are given in Bruning and Kintz (1987). Nonparametric tests were comprehensively described by Siegel (1956).

REVIEW QUESTIONS

1. List the parametric and nonparametric tests used for simple independent group and repeated measurement designs.
2. What is the purpose of these tests?
3. Why is the difference between groups not assessed solely on the basis of the difference between means?
4. What two measures determine the size of the *t* ratio?
5. How could each of the values be changed to increase the significance of the *t* ratio?
6. When can a one-tailed test be used? What is its purpose?
7. When must nonparametric tests be used instead of parametric tests?
8. Why is the Mann-Whitney Test less powerful than the *t*-test? Why is the Median Test less powerful than the Mann-Whitney Test?

CHAPTER

13

Statistical Analysis of Complex Group Designs

The parametric tests used for complex group designs have the same basic rationale as the *t*-tests used for simple group designs. The probability of chance differences is estimated in terms of the ratio of the difference between means to the variance of within-group or within-condition measures. For complex designs, the parametric test is called *analysis of variance*, usually abbreviated as ANOVA. The statistical ratio used for estimating the significance of the effects of independent variables is the *F* ratio. The larger the difference between means and the smaller the variance within groups or conditions, the larger will be the *F* ratio and the smaller the probability that the difference between groups is attributable to chance.

The requirements for simple designs regarding significance levels, normal distributions, equal variances, and the null hypothesis apply to complex group designs in the same way. The complexity of the statistical analysis varies according to the number of levels of each independent variable, the number of independent variables, and the extent to which there is a mixture of independent groups and repeated measures. ANOVAs are laborious to calculate with a pocket calculator, but computer programs for statistical calculations are readily available.

DESIGNS WITH MORE THAN TWO LEVELS OF ONE INDEPENDENT VARIABLE

Independent Groups

Where there are three or more levels of one independent variable, the parametric statistic is *simple analysis of variance*. As was the case for the *t*-test, slightly different calculations are required for independent groups and repeated measures. An example of a simple ANOVA for independent groups is a hypothetical study where three groups of brain damaged patients are required to name a set of 30 pictures. The independent variable is classification of the brain damaged patients, and has three levels—no aphasia, Broca's aphasia, and Wernicke's aphasia. The dependent variable is number of errors on the picture-naming test. To keep the example as simple as possible, there are only five patients in each group (Table 13–1). There appears to be a large difference among the means relative to the variance of scores within groups. This can be seen more easily by showing the data in distributed form (Table 13–2). The distribution of nonaphasic errors is considerably above those of the other two groups, which are closer together. The *F* ratio is calculated in terms of the difference between groups relative to the variance within groups. The results are shown in Table 13–3.

It is easy to see what contributes to the *F* ratio. The statistical analysis uses only the five error scores for each group. The *total variance* of the 15 scores is 529.40. This is *partitioned* into the *between group variance* (411.60) between the means of the three groups and the *within group*

TABLE 13–1.
Hypothetical Picture-Naming Error Scores for Three Independent Groups.

	Nonaphasic	Broca's Aphasia	Wernicke's Aphasia
	3	10	14
	5	13	16
	7	15	20
	8	17	23
	11	21	24
Mean Errors	6.8	15.2	19.4

TABLE 13–2.
Distributions of Picture-Naming Error Scores from Table 13–1.

Number of Naming Errors	Nonaphasic	Broca's	Wernicke's
1			
2			
3	x		
4			
5	x		
6			
7	x (M)		
8	x		
9			
10		x	
11	x		
12			
13		x	
14			x
15		x (M)	
16			x
17		x	
18			
19			(M)
20			x
21		x	
22			
23			x
24			x

variance (180.80) of the five scores within each group. Before calculating the F ratio, these *variance estimates* are made equivalent by dividing them by the *degrees of freedom* (df), which are 2 $(3 - 1)$ for between-group variance and 12 $[(5 - 1) + (5 - 1) + (5 - 1)]$ for within-group variance. The resulting mean square for between-group variance is divided by the

TABLE 13–3.
Simple ANOVA for Independent Groups.

Source of Variance	Sums of Squares	Degrees of Freedom (df)	Mean Squares	F
Between Groups	411.60	2	205.80	13.66
Within Groups	180.80	12	15.07	
Total	592.40	14		

mean square for within-group variance to get the F ratio of 13.66. This F ratio is significant beyond the .001 level for 2 and 12 degrees of freedom.

If the within-group variance remained the same, a larger difference between means would give a larger F ratio, and a smaller difference between means would give a smaller F ratio. If the difference between means remained the same, an increase in within-group variance would give a smaller F ratio and a decrease in within-group variance would give a larger F ratio. Thus, it is not difficult to understand how the probability of differences among groups is estimated in simple ANOVA for independent groups by partitioning the total variance into between-group and within-group variance.

Multiple Comparisons and Planned Comparisons between Pairs of Means

There remains another important step in the interpretation of significant differences among means for simple ANOVAs. Which of the means are significantly different from each other? The F ratio does not provide this information. It only indicates that there is a significant difference somewhere. Additional statistical tests are needed to determine the significance of differences between pairs of means. A series of t-tests might be carried out, but when a given mean is used in more than one test, the probability of chance differences becomes greater.

Where it is of interest to compare all pairs of means, *multiple comparison tests* are used. These tests, which are also called *post hoc comparisons*, *a posteriori comparisons*, or *supplemental computations*, adjust the within-group variance estimates to compensate for the greater probability of chance differences. The most common multiple comparison tests are the Tukey, Newman-Keuls, and Duncan tests. They are easily calculated, as they use mean differences, within-group variance estimates, and degrees of freedom from the ANOVA. Multiple comparisons can only be made when the F ratio is statistically significant. Calculation of the Newman-Keuls test for the previous data reveals that the nonaphasic patients made significantly fewer errors (.01 level) than the Broca's patients and the Wernicke's patients, but there was no significant difference even at the .05 level between the Broca's and Wernicke's patients.

These findings are confirmed by visual inspection of the distributions of scores of the three groups. The nonaphasic distribution was almost completely separated from the distributions of the two aphasic groups, and the distributions of Broca's and Wernicke's aphasics overlapped a great deal. However, exact probability estimates cannot be made by visual inspection of the data. The simple ANOVA in conjunction with multiple comparison tests provides a powerful statistical technique for estimating the probability of differences among three or more levels of one independent variable. Once again, the interpretation of significant differences as demonstrating the effect of the independent variable—natural groups—depends on how well other relevant variables were controlled.

An even more powerful technique for estimating the significance of differences among three or more levels of an independent variable can be used when the comparisons among means of greatest interest can be planned in advance. These *planned comparisons* must be based on exact predictions of mean differences made at the time the study is designed, prior to collecting the data. Because all possible pairs of means are not compared, the probability of chance differences does not increase as much for planned comparisons as for multiple comparisons, and a powerful test called the *Dunn Test* can be used to evaluate mean differences. Another great advantage of planned comparisons is that the F ratio does not have to be significant for the mean comparisons to be made.

Because much HCD research involves problems for which there is not enough knowledge for confident predictions to be made, multiple comparisons are used more than planned comparisons. In the present example, it would be of interest to compare all pairs of means by multiple comparison. However, researchers might feel confident enough of their past knowledge to predict that the nonaphasic group would score lowest and one aphasic group would score next lowest. In such a case, planned comparisons could be used to compare only two pairs of means.

Repeated Measurements

Although the calculations are different, the probability estimate for differences among three or more repeated measures is arrived at in essentially the same way as the probability estimate for three independent groups. The F ratio is calculated in terms of the ratio of between-condition and within-condition variance, and additional comparisons between means are calculated in about the same way as for independent groups.

Nonparametric Tests

Less powerful nonparametric tests making use of ranks or medians can be used to determine the significance of differences among three or more levels of one independent variable for both independent groups and repeated measures. These tests are not as useful as parametric tests, because additional comparisons of the significance of differences between pairs of means are not possible.

FACTORIAL DESIGNS

The next level of complexity of group designs involves factorial designs with two or more independent variables, each of which may have two or more levels. The parametric statistic used for the analysis of factorial designs is *factorial analysis of variance.*

In the simple ANOVA there is just one independent variable, and the ANOVA determines whether there is a significant difference between the three or more means. In factorial ANOVA, the significance of differences between means is determined for two or more independent variables. These tests of significance are called *main effects*, because they assess the effects of varying each of the independent variables. Interactions between the independent variables are also assessed.

Main Effects and Interactions

The most important difference between the simple and the factorial ANOVA is in the *interaction effects*, which do not occur in simple ANOVAs. Interactions are important for the purposes of the research design, because they indicate whether the effects of independent variables change at different levels of other independent variables.

Where there are two independent variables, two main effects and one interaction are assessed by the factorial ANOVA, as in the following example of a 2×3 independent group design:

Main Effects: Variable 1 – HCD (language disorder versus normal language)
Variable 2 – Age (5, 6, 7)
Interaction: HCD × Age

There is an interaction if the difference between language disordered and normal language groups changes for different age groups. This would occur if differences between language disordered and normal language groups were larger at age 5 than at age 7.

Where there are three independent variables, there are three main effects and four interactions, as in the following example of a 2x3x2 independent group design:

Main Effects: Variable 1 – HCD (2 levels)
Variable 2 – Age (3 levels)
Variable 3 – Sex (2 levels)
Interactions: HCD × Age
HCD × Sex
Age × Sex
HCD × Age × Sex

Interactions between two variables could occur in the same way as in the previous example. An HCD × Age × Sex interaction would occur if the HCD x Age interaction was different for male subjects and female subjects. This would occur if there was a smaller difference between groups with language disorders and normal language groups at ages 6 and 7 than at age 5 for female subjects, but only at age 7 for male subjects.

Where there are four independent variables, there are four main effects, and now there are 11 interactions, as in the following example of a 2×3×2×3 mixed design:

Main Effects: Variable 1 – HCD
                 Variable 2 – Age
                 Variable 3 – Sex
                 Variable 4 – Language Level (Lexical, Syntactic, Semantic)

Interactions: HCD × Age
                 HCD × Sex
                 HCD × Language Level
                 Age × Sex
                 Age × Language Level
                 Sex × Language Level

                 HCD × Age × Sex
                 HCD × Age × Language Level
                 HCD × Sex × Language Level
                 Age × Sex × Language Level

                 HCD × Age × Sex × Language Level

Interactions among three variables would occur in the same way as in the previous example. The most complex interaction could occur if younger male subjects were equally impaired at all levels and older male subjects were only impaired at the syntactic and semantic levels, whereas younger female subjects were only impaired at the syntactic and semantic levels and older female subjects only at the semantic level. Such findings could have important implications for diagnosis and intervention. Even aside from the problems of finding the 180 to 360 subjects needed to fill the 36 cells of the design, however, the statistical calculations and the interpretation of the interactions become more complex as more independent variables are added.

Error Terms: Within-Group and Within-Condition Variance

F ratios for main effects and interactions in factorial ANOVAs are calculated in the same manner as F ratios in simple ANOVAs. The magnitude of the differences between means is related to the magnitude of variance within groups or conditions. The larger the difference between means and the smaller the variance within groups or conditions, the larger the F ratio and the smaller the probability that the mean differences occurred by chance. Within-group and within-condition variances are called *error terms*, because they are the estimates of error against which mean differences are evaluated.

The error term in simple ANOVAs is easily identified, because the total variance is partitioned into only two components, the between group/condition and the within group/condition variance. In factorial ANOVAs the choice of error term is more complicated, as the total variance is divided into many more components, and great care must be taken to select the appropriate error term for each F ratio. The procedures for selecting error terms are described in statistic texts, and the computer programs used for factorial ANOVAs usually select appropriate error terms.

AN EXAMPLE OF FACTORIAL ANALYSIS OF VARIANCE

A relatively simple example of factorial ANOVA using fewer than the minimum number of subjects per cell will indicate how main effects and interactions are calculated and interpreted. The example uses a 2×3 mixed factorial design having two independent variables, one with two levels and the other with three levels. The subjects are adults with acquired sensorineural hearing loss. The first independent variable is age, with two independent groups of five young adults and five older adults. The second independent variable is amount of training in speechreading, with repeated measurements of the same subjects after 0, 8, and 16 hours of training the subjects to use speechreading cues. The dependent variable is percent of words correctly repeated on alternate forms of a test for repeating spoken words presented face-to-face. The order of presentation of the alternate tests is randomized. The purpose of the study is to determine whether different amounts of speechreading training may be needed for persons of different ages.

The percent of words correctly repeated by individual subjects at each stage of training is shown in Table 13–4.

The basic data obtained with this factorial design are three scores for each of the five subjects in each of the two groups. From these 15 scores are calculated the measures of central tendency and variability used in the factorial ANOVA (more subjects would be needed if this were a real study).

The 2×3 ANOVA assesses the statistical significance of the two main effects for age and amount of training, plus the interaction between age and amount of training. The main effect for the between-group variable

TABLE 13–4.
Percent of Words Correctly Repeated.

| | | Younger Subjects | | | | Older Subjects | | |
| | | Hours of Training | | | | Hours of Training | | |
	0	8	16	Mean	0	8	16	Mean
	55	76	92	74	50	60	68	59
	68	85	96	83	62	71	83	72
	42	63	85	63	46	55	68	56
	21	87	93	67	20	33	42	32
	35	74	82	64	30	40	48	39
Means	44	77	90	70	42	52	62	52
Means of Combined Groups					43	64	76	

of age is shown by the mean for each group, 70 percent correct for the younger subjects and only 52 percent correct for the older subjects. The main effect for the repeated measurement of hours of training is the mean of the combined groups, 43 percent for 0 hours, 64 percent for 8 hours, and 76 percent for 16 hours, a steady improvement with training.

It is important to note that the main effect for one independent variable is obtained by *pooling* the levels of the other independent variable. The main effect for age is obtained by pooling the results of the three amounts of training, and the main effect for training is obtained by pooling the two ages.

The researchers' interest is not confined to main effects. They not only wish to determine if there is a significant difference in performance with age (main effect for age) and an improvement with practice (main effect for hours of training), but whether both groups improve at the same rate. This important information is indicated by the interaction of age and hours of training. The interaction can be seen by comparing the change in the means of the two groups at each stage of training, as shown in Figure 13.1.

There is an apparent interaction. Both groups begin training at about the same level of accuracy, but the younger subjects improve much more than the older. The study appears to have resulted in interesting and important findings. However, the amount of within-group variance associated with each mean is not shown. It is necessary to statistically analyze the data to demonstrate that the observed trends have not occurred by chance.

Results of the ANOVA

The results of the ANOVA for the 2×3 mixed factorial design are shown in Table 13–5.

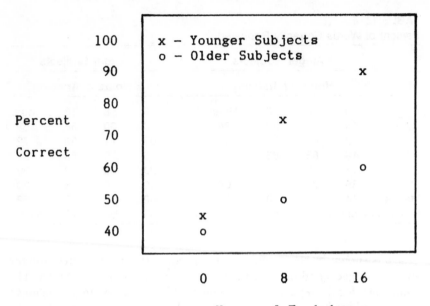

FIGURE 13.1. Interaction between Age and Amount of Training.

Table 13–5 is organized differently than the simple ANOVA table (Table 13–3). The sums of squares are omitted, and the level of significance (p) of the F ratios is given. The main effect of age is not significant at the .05 level (where the symbol points to the right [p >] it means "probability greater than," and where it points to the left [p <] it means "probability less than"). Although there was a large difference between the group means, the distributions of the scores of the small groups overlapped. The main effect for hours of training was significant beyond the .01 level. Performance of the two groups averaged together improved with training. The

TABLE 13–5.
Results of the ANOVA for the 2×3 Mixed Factorial Design.

Source of Variance	df	Mean Squares	F	p
Age (A)	1	2576	5.18	(p > .05)
Hours of Training (T)	2	2776	44.80	(p < .01)
Age × Training Interaction (AT)	2	480	7.75	(p < .01)
Error Term for A	8	498		
Error Term for T and AT	16	62		

tion of groups and training was significant beyond the .01 level, apparently because the younger subjects improved more with training.

The Source of Variance column in Table 13–5 has more entries than the simple ANOVA table (Table 13–3), where only the between-group and within-group variance contribute to the total variance. In the factorial ANOVA, the F ratio is still calculated in terms of the ratio of between group/condition and within group/condition variance. For age, there is a large mean square because a large proportion of the total variance is attributable to the large difference between the group means (70 and 52), but there is also a relatively large variance between subjects within groups (Error Term for A). The error term is based on the variance between subjects with the variance between age groups removed. Thus, the F ratio for age is based on the same type of ratio of between-group and within-group variance as the t-test.

The F ratio for the main effect of training is calculated according to the same rationale. There is a large mean square for training because much of the total variance is attributable to the large mean differences between hours of training for combined groups (43, 64, and 76). The F ratio is calculated by comparing the variance among the mean hours of training for the combined groups to the relatively small variance among training conditions for each subject with the variance between training conditions removed (Error Term for T and AT). This variance was small because each subject improved from 0 to 8 and from 8 to 16 hours.

The F ratio for the interaction is most easily understood in terms of *residual variance*. There is a total variance among the means for each training period for each group. The variance among these six means can be partitioned into the variance of the two main effects and the interaction. The two main effects were quite large and took up a large proportion of the total variance, as shown by their large mean squares. The variance among the six means not attributable to the differences between age groups and among training conditions is the residual variance attributable to the interaction of groups and training conditions.

The residual variance can be seen by examining the graphic representation of the interaction in Figure 13.1. If the difference between groups had been exactly the same for all three training conditions, there would have been no residual variance and no interaction. All of the variance among the six means would have been attributable to the two main effects. However, there was a very small difference between groups at 0 hours training and a very large difference at 16 hours training. This residual variance resulted in a significant interaction between the two independent variables of age and amount of training.

It is important to understand the concept of partitioning variance into components and the concept of residual variance, as they apply to the calculation of all interactions in factorial designs. In factorial designs with more than two independent variables, there are many more interactions, but the partitioning of variance among main effects and interactions occurs in the same way.

Interpretation of Main Effect and Interaction

Where an interaction is significant, the main effects need not be interpreted, because they are explained by the interaction. This can be seen in the present study. The main effect of groups was not of primary interest because it involved a comparison of group means pooled across hours of training, and the main effect of hours of training was not of primary interest because it compared means pooled across groups. If the interaction had not been significant, however, significant main effects would provide useful information about the effects of age and training.

Multiple Comparisons and Planned Comparisons

If the interaction had not been significant, additional computations would have been needed to interpret the significant main effect of training, because the significant F ratio does not indicate which of the differences among the three means were significant. A multiple comparison test of the type described for the simple ANOVA is needed. A Tukey test revealed that the scores of the pooled groups increased significantly (.01 level) from 0 to 8 hours training and from 8 to 16 hours training.

In a study like the present one, the significant interaction can be interpreted by inspecting the pattern of mean differences. It can be concluded that the younger subjects were only slightly better than the older subjects before training began, but showed greater improvement with training. If the trends had been less clear, however, further statistical analysis would be needed. A multiple comparison test would make all possible comparisons among the six means, with the error term adjusted to compensate for the increased probability of chance differences.

A Tukey test was used as the test for multiple comparisons. There was a significant increase (.01 level) in scores for the younger group from 0 to 8 hours training, but the increase from 8 to 16 hours was not significant. For the older group, only the increase from 0 to 16 hours was significant (.01 level). The differences between the two groups were significant (.01 level) at both 8 and 16 hours, but not at 0 hours. The remaining comparisons were between groups at different hours of training. The only comparisons of interest revealed that the mean for the older group was significantly higher (.05 level) at 16 hours but not at 8 hours than the mean for the young group at 0 hours training.

The multiple comparisons provide a great deal of information. Both groups significantly improved during training, but at different rates. At the beginning they were not significantly different, but the younger group obtained significantly larger scores than the older group after training had begun. The older group did not significantly exceed the younger group's pretraining scores until they had 16 hours of training. The extent to which this information is used depends on the purpose of the study. If the researchers want only to assess the progress of each group separately or to compare groups at each stage of training, more powerful planned comparisons could be used. If, in addition to these comparisons, they also wanted to compare one group at one stage of training with the other group at another stage of training, multiple comparisons would be necessary.

The choice of the method for additional statistical comparisons of interactions illustrates the close relationship between the exact purpose of the study and the data analysis. If, on the basis of previous research, the researchers had decided that the purpose of the research was to assess the progress of each group and to compare groups at each stage, only these planned comparisons of the means would be made. The increased statistical power would permit a more sensitive test of the training effects for each group.

When the present data were analyzed by planned comparisons of the training effects for each group, the increased statistical power revealed a significant increase in the scores of the young group from 0 to 8 hours (.01 level) but not from 8 to 16 hours ($p > .05$). This result had also been found with the multiple comparisons. However, the planned comparisons revealed a significant increase (.01 level) in the older group's scores from 0 to 8 hours and from 8 to 16 hours. Inspection of the individual scores indicates that the lack of significant increase from 8 to 16 hours for the younger group was the result of a ceiling effect. After 16 hours of training, the younger subjects approached perfect scores on the word repetition test. This finding, which was not revealed as clearly by the multiple comparison test, would be important for planning further research. If more training were to be given, more difficult tests would be needed for valid comparisons of the proficiency of younger and older subjects.

Planned comparisons are most useful when researchers have enough prior knowledge to decide on very specific purposes, and multiple comparisons are most useful when the researchers must rely more on guesswork concerning the outcome of the research. For the present example, the choice of the method of additional comparisons would depend on the amount and type of previous knowledge of researchers and practitioners about auditory training.

Relationship between Factorial ANOVA and Other Research Events

This relatively simple factorial ANOVA is an excellent example of how all research events are interrelated. The results of the ANOVA could not be fully interpreted without reference to the purpose of the experiment.

The factorial design could have served many different purposes. At least five separate studies were nested in the 2×3 design. The older and younger subjects could be compared for three different amounts of training, the equivalent of three separate independent group designs. The three training conditions could be assessed for each group, the equivalent of two single-factor repeated measure designs. Putting all of these separate designs together in one factorial design permitted a detailed comparison of the interactive effects of the two independent variables.

A MORE COMPLEX FACTORIAL DESIGN

An example of a factorial design with three independent variables will indicate how ANOVAs involving more than one interaction are analyzed and interpreted. To keep the example as simple and clear as possible, a somewhat artificial hypothetical study is used, with fewer than the minimum number of subjects per cell.

Assume that the researchers want to find out whether developmental language disorders are associated with (not "caused by") deficient functioning of the left cerebral hemisphere. The left hemisphere seems to subserve language processes in most normal right-handed individuals (note cautious terminology). Tests called *dichotic listening tests* show that when different linguistic stimuli are presented simultaneously to the two ears, recognition accuracy tends to be best for the right ear, which has its strongest connections to the left cerebral hemisphere; and when different nonlinguistic stimuli such as environmental sounds are presented simultaneously to the two ears, recognition accuracy tends to be best for the left ear, which has its strongest connections to the right cerebral hemisphere.

The researchers decide to attack the problem of whether the "language" hemisphere of right-handed children with language disorders is functioning normally by giving them a test where pairs of one-syllable words are presented simultaneously to the two ears. If they do not perform better with the right ear, it might indicate that their left hemisphere is not performing properly. This study could be done with a simple repeated measure design with two levels of one independent variable (ears). However, proving no difference would require accepting the null hypothesis. This would be inadvisable. Among other reasons, there might be no difference because the test was not sensitive enough to show the effect.

To control for test sensitivity and provide a better means of interpreting a lack of difference between ears, the researchers could also test a control group of right-handed non-disordered children. If the non-disordered children showed the expected right ear superiority and the children who are language disordered did not, it would suggest a difference in the functioning of the left hemisphere of the children who are language disordered. This design would be a 2×2 factorial design with two independent variables, one involving two independent groups (children with and without language disorders) and the other involving repeated measurement of the two ears. The researchers would predict a significant interaction of ears and groups, where the normal children showed right ear superiority but the children who are language disordered did not.

To rule out the possibility that the deficiency of the children who are language disordered involved both cerebral hemispheres, the researchers could give another test for the recognition of pairs of environmental sounds presented to the two ears. The children who are language disordered should have the same left ear superiority as the normal children on this task, indicating normal functioning of the "nonlanguage" hemisphere. If only the nonverbal test were given to the two groups and both had a left-ear advantage, a 2×2 mixed factorial ANOVA would show a main effect for ears but no interaction between ears and groups.

A design where both the verbal and the nonverbal tests are given to both groups combines two 2×2 factorial designs. In the design involving the verbal test, the researchers expect a significant interaction, but in the design involving the nonverbal test, they do not expect a significant interaction. Putting the two designs together makes a 2×2×2 mixed factorial design. If, as expected, there were a groups × ears interaction for the verbal task but not for the nonverbal task, there could be a significant interaction of groups × ears × tasks. The purpose of this example is to show that such complex interactions, which may occur more often than simple interactions in HCDs, can be interpreted in as simple and logical a manner as simple interactions.

The minimum number of subjects for the eight cells of the 2×2×2 design would be 40 to 80. In this hypothetical study only eight subjects were used, to simplify the interpretation of the raw data. Significant effects occurred because the artificial data were created to exhibit very consistent trends. The two groups of four right-handed subjects were matched on relevant variables. Each subject was given both tests, with the order of tests counterbalanced.

The percentage of correct responses of individual subjects for each ear on each task is shown in Table 13–6.

Table 13–6 contains all the information needed for calculation of the ANOVA and the descriptive statistics used for the interpretation of the ANOVA. The scores of individual subjects are given in four columns, and include one score for each ear on each test. These 32 scores are the raw data obtained with the 2×2×2 factorial design. The factorial ANOVA partitions the variance among these 32 scores to obtain the between-means variance estimates and the error terms for the main effects and interactions.

TABLE 13-6.
Hypothetical Results for a Factorial Design with Three Independent Variables.

| | Word Test | | Sound Test | |
	Right Ear	Left Ear	Right Ear	Left Ear
Normal	73	45	44	85
Language	84	37	36	77
	86	36	34	84
	75	45	43	75
Language	37	46	45	75
Disorder	46	34	33	84
	35	36	43	72
	46	44	45	85

The trends can be seen by looking at the individual test scores. The normal subjects scored consistently higher on the right ear on the words task and on the left ear on the sounds task. The subjects who are language disordered showed the same trend as the subjects who are not on the sounds task, but no consistent ear difference on the words task. The comparisons between groups can be summarized by noting that they differed on only one of four repeated measures, the right ear score on the words task. This one difference will lead to a significant groups × ears × tasks interaction. The interaction could be interpreted as suggesting that children who are language disordered have a specific deficit in left-hemisphere functioning.

The means for the various conditions are the descriptive statistics needed to interpret the main effects and interactions. The means that indicate the main effects and interactions are shown in Table 13-7.

The means are similar because the data were created to show the complex interactions in as clear a manner as possible. The trends of greatest interest are shown by the group × ear × task means. The normal language group has a right ear advantage for words and a left ear advantage for sounds. The language disorder group has a left ear advantage for sounds but no difference between ears for words.

Results of the ANOVA

For simplicity, the ANOVA table has been condensed in Table 13-8. All of the main effects and interactions are significant beyond the .01 level. Where a higher-order interaction is significant, it is unnecessary to interpret the main effects and lower-order interactions. In the present study, all of the information concerning the effects of the independent variables

TABLE 13-7.
Means Showing Main Effects and Interactions for Data in Table 13-6.

Combined mean for all subjects (all scores pooled)			55
Group means (pooled ears and tasks)		Normal Language	60
		Language Disorder	50
Ear means (pooled groups and tasks)		Right Ear	50
		Left Ear	60
Task means (pooled groups and ears)		Dichotic Words	50
		Dichotic Sounds	60
Group × Ear means (pooled tasks)		Normal: Right Ear	59
		Left Ear	61
		Disorder: Right Ear	41
		Left Ear	60
Group × Task means (pooled ears)		Normal: Words	60
		Sounds	60
		Disorder: Words	41
		Sounds	60
Ear × Task means (pooled groups)		Words: Right Ear	60
		Left Ear	40
		Sounds: Right Ear	40
		Left Ear	80
Group × Ear × Task means	Normal:	Words: Right Ear	80
		Left Ear	41
		Sounds: Right Ear	39
		Left Ear	80
	Disorder:	Words: Right Ear	41
		Left Ear	40
		Sounds: Right Ear	42
		Left Ear	79

is contained in the means for the GET interaction. Because each independent variable had only two levels, no additional comparisons are needed. Both groups had a left ear advantage on the sounds task, but only the normal language group had a right ear advantage on the words task. This finding confirms the prediction that subjects who are language disordered would not show evidence of left hemisphere dominance for language.

Although the significant GET interaction contains all of the necessary information about the study, it is useful to interpret all main effects and interactions with reference to studies where the highest order interaction is not significant. As each of the main effects had only two levels of the independent variable, the significant effects can be directly interpreted without multiple comparison tests. The significant main effects for groups (means of 60 for the normal language group and 50 for the language

TABLE 13–8.
Summary of Analysis of Variance.

Source	df	F
Groups (G)	1	25.20*
Ears (E)	1	25.03*
Tasks (T)	1	75.10*
GE	1	19.56*
GT	1	81.00*
ET	1	145.90*
GET	1	13.97*

* p < .01

disorder group), tasks (50 for the words task and 60 for the sounds task), and ears (50 for the right ear and 60 for the left ear) were all attributable to the lower right ear scores of the language disorder group on the words task.

The significant lower-order interactions were also attributable to the lower right ear word score for the language disorder group (Table 13–9). In the first two interactions there would be no interaction if the one mean were not lower. In the third interaction there would be an even larger interaction between words and tasks if the right ear word score of the language disorder group had been the same as that for the normal language group. The right ear word mean would have been 80, and the ear × task interaction would have involved a complete reversal.

The interpretations of main effects and interactions are rendered unnecessary by the significant higher-order interaction (Table 13–10). The normal language group shows the expected reversal of right and left ear

TABLE 13–9.
Lower-Order Interactions.

Group × Ear Interaction		Right Ear	Left Ear
	Normal Language	59	61
	Language Disorder	41	60
Group × Task Interaction		Words	Sounds
	Normal Language	60	60
	Language Disorder	41	60
Ear × Task Interaction		Right Ear	Left Ear
	Words	60	40
	Sounds	40	80

TABLE 13–10.
High-Order Interaction between Groups, Ears, and Tasks.

	NORMAL LANGUAGE			LANGUAGE DISORDER	
	Right Ear	Left Ear		Right Ear	Left Ear
Words	80	41	Words	41	40
Sounds	39	80	Sounds	42	79

scores for the two tasks. If this were a study of normal subjects only, there would have been a highly significant interaction between tasks and ears. The language disorder group did not have this reversal, as there were no ear differences on the words task. If this were a study of subjects who are language disordered alone, they might still have had a significant interaction between ears and tasks, but it would have been smaller than that for the normal group. The interaction of group × task × ear occurred because of a predicted but relatively subtle difference between the tasks × ears interactions of the two groups.

Interpretation

Like the simpler 2×3 factorial design, the 2×2×2 design is very thorough. It partitions the variance of the 32 numbers arising from the four scores for the eight subjects into main effects and interactions and isolates the effect of interest in the higher-order interaction. As before, the interpretation of the analysis depends on the adequacy of the design and procedure, as well as the exact purposes of the research.

The data of this artificial study were carefully selected to produce trends that could be easily interpreted. For an actual study, 20 to 40 subjects per group would be needed to fulfill the minimum requirement of 5 to 10 subjects per cell. Ear differences would not be uniform, as dichotic tests are open to many sources of difficulty. Assuming that all of the potential design and procedural problems had been solved, the study would indicate that certain verbal stimuli were not processed efficiently by the left cerebral hemisphere of language disordered children. Further research would be needed to determine the implications for intervention.

NON-PARAMETRIC TESTS FOR FACTORIAL DESIGNS

There are no nonparametric tests for factorial designs that permit the assessment of interactions.

OTHER ANALYSES OF VARIANCE

Two additional procedures for analyzing the results of complex designs, analysis of covariance (ANCOVA) and multivariate analysis of variance (MANOVA), are discussed in the next chapter. They both involve correlational analysis as well as analysis of variance.

ADDITIONAL INFORMATION

Statistical analyses of complex group designs are discussed in advanced statistics texts, with especially clear explanations given by Edwards (1985), Hays (1981), and Keppel (1982).

REVIEW QUESTIONS

1. Why are additional statistical tests needed for simple analysis of variance?
2. How is the total variance partitioned in simple ANOVA?
3. What determines the size of the F ratio in simple ANOVA?
4. What is the difference between multiple comparisons and planned comparisons in simple ANOVA?
5. What determines whether multiple comparisons or planned comparisons will be used to interpret simple ANOVA?
6. What is meant by the term *residual variance* in factorial ANOVA?

EXERCISES (answers are given in Appendix D)

1. List the main effects and interactions for each of the following designs:
   a. Effectiveness of two hearing aids for speech discrimination in quiet and noise.
   b. Effects of age, sex, and speaking task (picture description versus story retelling) on articulation errors of children without HCDs.
   c. Effects of age, education, amount of training, and amount of hearing impairment on speechreading in adults with sensorineural loss.
2. Give an example of a significant interaction that might occur for the highest-order interaction in each of the three designs listed in Exercise 1.

CHAPTER
14

Statistical Analysis of Relationships

This chapter is concerned with methods for analyzing relationships in correlation designs and in combined correlation and group designs. Relationships are evaluated in estimating the degree of *covariance* or *nonindependence* of variables in correlation designs. When two or more variables are assessed for the same group of subjects, the variables covary or are nonindependent to the extent that changes in one variable tend to be accompanied by changes in the other variable. The *correlation* between variables is usually expressed in terms of a *correlation coefficient* that varies between 1.00 and −1.00. A high correlation or strong relationship can be either positive or negative. A positive correlation, for example, between height and weight, would tend to approach 1.00, and a negative correlation, for example, between age and reaction time in children, would tend to approach −1.00. Where there is no relationship, that is, the two variables are independent, the correlation would tend to approach .00.

Correlations can serve as a basis for predictions. The higher the correlation between the predicting and the predicted variable, the better the

135

prediction. The term *regression* is used to describe the estimation or prediction of one variable by another variable. This aspect of the analysis of relationships can have practical importance for HCDs, if an HCD can be predicted by a particular variable or set of variables.

As discussed previously, the limitation of information about relationships is that covariation, correlation, and regression cannot be used as proof that a change in one variable has caused a change in another variable. Covariation is only one of the three conditions required for the demonstration of causality. The other two conditions are that the change in one variable preceded the change in the other variable, and that plausible alternative causal variables have been ruled out. The latter condition is difficult to achieve in research involving the statistical analysis of relationships. If a strong relationship is found between two variables it is always possible that both variables are correlated with a third variable. It is very difficult to reach definite conclusions on the basis of correlational analysis alone. Therefore, correlational analyses are often used in conjunction with other types of data analyses.

Statistical analyses of relationships range from simple and easily understood correlations between two variables to complex multivariate correlation analyses. Some of the most representative forms of correlation analysis will be briefly described here. All correlation analyses are based on the reasoning used to interpret simple correlations and partial correlations. It is important, therefore, to thoroughly understand simple correlations and partial correlations.

SIMPLE CORRELATIONS OF TWO VARIABLES

A simple correlation estimates the degree of relationship, that is, the amount of covariance, of two variables. A hypothetical study in which scores were obtained on two different speech discrimination tests for 10 subjects can be used as an example. The pairs of scores are repeated measurements of the same subjects, expressed as percent correct, as shown in Table 14–1. In this set of data, subjects tend to have about the same score on both tests. This can be seen in a two-dimensional *scatter plot*, where the Test 1 score of each subject is plotted on the vertical scale and the Test 2 score is plotted on the horizontal scale (Figure 14.1). The scatter plot shows that high scores on one test *tend to be* accompanied by high scores on the other. Scores on the two tests are positively correlated. The strength of the tendency for a positive relationship is expressed by the correlation coefficient.

The most powerful test for simple correlations is a parametric test called the *Pearson product moment correlation*. The correlation coefficient,

TABLE 14-1.
Hypothetical Results for Two Speech
Discrimination Tests.

Subject	Test 1	Test 2
1	95	90
2	86	93
3	90	88
4	73	77
5	65	74
6	78	80
7	86	95
8	82	80
9	87	87
10	72	65

which is denoted by r, is based on the degree of covariance of the pairs of scores relative to the variance within each set of scores. The greater the proportion of the total variance of the scores attributable to covariance, the higher will be the correlation. In calculating the correlation, the estimate of covariance is divided by the estimate of within-test variance.

In the present example, $r = .81$, indicating a strong relationship between the two tests. The proportion of total variance attributable to covariance is determined by squaring the correlation coefficient. Where $r = .81$, $r^2 = .66$. This indicates the amount of variance that the two tests have in common. In this example, 66 percent of the variance in the scores of each test is related to the variance of the other test. To this extent, they are both measuring the same thing.

The correlation coefficient indicates the degree of relationship, but does not demonstrate that the correlation could not have occurred by chance. The statistical significance of correlations, like the statistical significance of differences between measures, is expressed in terms of the .05 or .01 level of confidence, as determined from tables. The significance depends on the size of the correlation and the number of subjects. Where there are only five subjects, a correlation coefficient has to be .878 to be significant at the .05 level and .959 to be significant at the .01 level. Where there are 100 subjects, the coefficient only has to be .195 for the .05 level and .254 for the .01 level.

If two variables were perfectly correlated, the scores would fall along a diagonal line, as in Figure 14.2. The correlation coefficients would approach 1.00 or −1.00, and r^2 would approach 100 percent, demonstrating that the two variables are perfectly related.

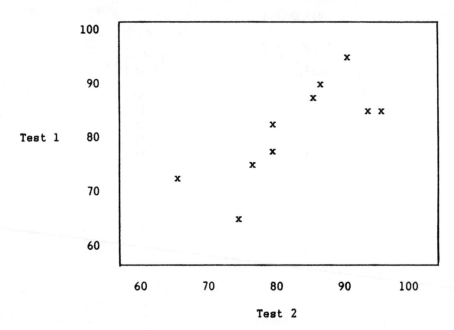

FIGURE 14.1. Scatter Plot of Speech Discrimination Test Scores.

If there was no relationship between the scores on the two tests, the scatter plot would show an equal distribution of scores (Figure 14.3). With such a perfect lack of correlation, both r and r^2 would approach .00. All of the variance would be attributable to variance within each set of measures, and none to covariance of the measures. The two measures could be said to be *independent*. However, conclusions concerning the independence of two variables on the basis of nonsignificant correlations greater than .00 should be made with great caution.

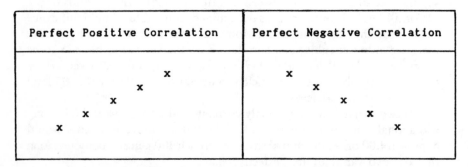

FIGURE 14.2. Hypothetical Scatter Plots.

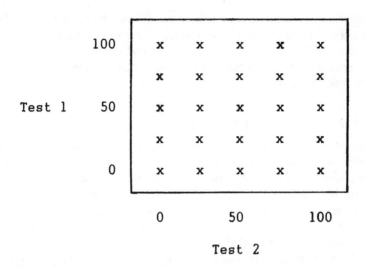

FIGURE 14.3. Hypothetical Scatter Plot of Uncorrelated Variables.

Low correlations can only be interpreted as indications of the independence of variables when both variables are adequately distributed. Where there are ceiling or floor effects (see Chapter 10), as in the following extreme examples, correlations will be low because one variable is relatively invariant. In such cases, it would be wrong to conclude that the variables are independent (Figure 14.4). Where there is a ceiling or a floor effect, any relationship that might exist is decreased by the upper or lower

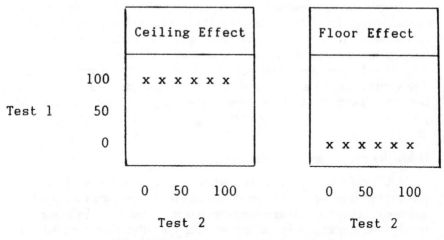

FIGURE 14.4. Hypothetical Scatter Plots.

limit of the distribution. Where there are ceiling effects, a more difficult test is needed to reach conclusions about the independence of variables, and when there are floor effects, an easier test is needed. This is one of the reasons why the distribution of scores should always be examined in interpreting HCD research.

Interpretation of Simple Correlations

Simple correlations can be interpreted in several ways, depending on the purpose of the research. In the previous example, the correlation between alternate forms of a speech discrimination test could serve as an index of the *reliability* of the test. If one test were given in the clinic and the other test given under real-life listening conditions, the correlation could serve as an index of the *external validity* of the clinic test in predicting speech discrimination in real-life situations.

Whatever the interpretation of correlations, they apply only to the sample of subjects for whom the measures were obtained. For correlations as well as group designs, there is a problem of generalizing the results for a given sample of subjects to the entire population from which the sample was obtained. The recommended procedure is to *replicate* the findings by determining the correlation between measures for another group of subjects.

If the correlations involve a measure with questionable validity, such as a test of syntactic ability, it is also useful to estimate the extent to which the findings can generalize to another measure of the same ability. This can be done by determining the correlation between the measure in question and another measure of the same ability, preferably a measure that has external validity. For example, scores on a syntax test might be correlated with the correctness of syntax in everyday conversations.

Simple correlations can be very useful for prediction, and also as tools for estimating the reliability and validity of measures. The main precaution regarding the interpretation of correlations is that they should not be taken at face value. It is advisable to replicate the findings with different subjects and different measures before making practical use of the findings. The samples should always be as large as possible, as small samples are not very informative. These precautions apply to all correlational procedures.

Other Tests of Simple Correlations

Like other parametric tests, certain assumptions are made for the product moment correlation test. The scores have to be evenly distributed, and the relationship between measures has to be *linear*. To be linear, the trend of the scatter plot has to be a straight line rather than a curved line.

If these two assumptions are not met, the correlation coefficient may not give a valid indication of the relationship between measures.

Nonparametric tests of correlation avoid problems of distribution and linearity. A common nonparametric test for simple correlations is the *Spearman rank-difference correlation*. The scores for each variable are ranked. The correlation coefficient, which is called *Rho* or *R*, is calculated on the basis of the difference between ranks. The smaller the differences between the pairs of ranks, the higher the correlation. Where each subject's ranks tend to be the same for both measures, there will be small differences and a high positive correlation. High negative correlations occur when a high rank on one measure tends to be accompanied by a low rank on the other measure. Because of the conversion of scores to ranks, the nonparametric test is less powerful than the product moment test of correlation.

Point biserial correlation determines the relationship between two variables where one variable is divided into two categories and the other is normally distributed. An example would be the relationship between a pass or fail score on a clinical test and age. The *Phi coefficient* determines the relationship between two variables when both are scored in only two categories, such as pass and fail. Because of the conversion of scores to categories, these tests are much less powerful than the Spearman rank-difference test.

Intercorrelations among Three or More Variables

A major limitation in the information obtained by correlation designs is that the correlation between two variables may be attributable to their joint correlations with other variables. This prevents any definite conclusions about the effect of one variable on the other. The same limitation applies to group designs that attempt to prove that a change in a dependent variable was caused by the independent variable and not by an uncontrolled variable.

An obvious way to determine the effects of uncontrolled variables is to calculate correlations between all relevant variables. Unfortunately, the intercorrelations among all relevant variables do not provide enough information by themselves. More complex correlational analyses are needed to assess the relationships among relevant variables. These analyses will be described in the following sections. In the early stages of research, however, it may be of interest to examine the intercorrelations to suggest the direction of further research. For example, where relevant uncontrolled variables such as age and education are found to be correlated with the variables that are being studied, such as syntactic ability, researchers know that the variables must be controlled in further research.

PARTIAL CORRELATION

When two variables are found to be correlated, it is often necessary to rule out the possibility that the relationship is attributable to their joint correlation with a third variable. The effect of the third variable can be "partialled out" by a very simple procedure called *partial correlation*. For example, there are three variables called A, B, and C, and the researchers are interested in the relationship between A (e.g., age) and B (e.g., amount of improvement in speechreading with 16 hours of training) independent of their joint relationship with C (amount of hearing loss). The correlations between A and B, A and C, and B and C are calculated. Then a simple formula is used to adjust the correlation between A and B to eliminate the influence of their joint correlation with C.

If there is a high negative correlation (e.g., −.90) between age (A) and amount of improvement with speechreading training (B), the researchers might conclude that learning ability decreases as a function of age. However, the relationship of age and improvement might be attributable to their joint correlation with amount of hearing loss (C). Where the joint correlations with the third variable are also high (e.g., .90 between age and hearing loss and −.90 between amount of improvement and hearing loss), removing their effects by partial correlation will greatly reduce the correlation between improvement and age (from −.90 to −.47) and the amount of common variance will be greatly reduced (from 81 percent to 22 percent). Where the joint correlations with the third variable are lower (e.g., .70 and −.70), the reduction in the correlation (−.90 to −.80) and in the common variance (81 percent to 64 percent) is not as great.

Partial correlation seems to be a very useful technique for estimating the unique relationship between two variables. In the previous example, other correlated variables such as visual acuity could also be partialled out to approach a causal explanation of the relationship between age and improvement with training. Some of the complex correlational procedures that will be described do use a form of partial correlation to estimate unique relationships between variables.

As with all correlational procedures, however, partial correlations may be difficult to interpret. In the present example, it is not easy to determine which should be the relationship of interest. It may be as important to determine the relation of hearing loss to improvement with training as it is to determine the relationship between age and improvement. It is easy to become confused. Partial correlations should only be used when the exact purpose is clear.

The information sought from partial correlations might also be obtained from a complex group design with age, amount of hearing loss, and amount of training as independent variables. Then the interrelationship among variables could be interpreted in terms of the interaction of age × hearing loss × training. Thus, the same problem could be investigated using two different types of design. The choice of design would depend on the exact purpose of the research plus practical considerations such as the number and type of available subjects. Yet another way of approaching this particular problem would be to use a design that combines group and correlation designs, analysis of covariance, which will be described in a later section of this chapter.

MULTIPLE CORRELATION

Instead of being interested in the relationship between two variables, researchers may wish to determine the relationship of one variable (e.g., amount of improvement with speechreading training) to a number of other variables (e.g., age, hearing impairment, education). *Multiple correlation* is a procedure for calculating the correlation between one variable and two or more other variables. The single variable is called the *criterion variable*, and can be considered the dependent variable. The multiple variables are called *predictor variables* and can be considered independent variables. Instead of partialling out the separate correlations of each predictor variable with the criterion variable, the joint relationship between the predictor (independent) variables and the criterion (dependent) variable is calculated.

In the examples used for partial correlation it was of interest to evaluate the relationship between age and improvement where the effects of hearing loss had been removed. If the purpose were to use all possible variables to help predict amount of success in speechreading training, a high correlation (e.g., −.90) between amount of improvement and age might be sufficient by itself. If, however, there were a lower correlation (e.g., −.70) between age and amount of improvement, other predictor variables might be sought. Additional predictor variables will increase the correlation to the extent that their correlation with the criterion variable is high, and their correlations with the other predictor variables are low. Where hearing loss is also correlated −.70 with improvement, the multiple correlation increases from −.70 (49 percent common variance) to −.81 (65 percent common variance) when the second predictor variable (hearing loss) is correlated .50 with the first predictor variable (age), and only from .70 to .77 (59 percent common variance) when the second predictor variable is correlated .70 with the first predictor variable. Additional predictor variables would increase the multiple correlation to the extent that they were highly correlated with the criterion variable and were not highly correlated with the other predictor variables.

Multiple correlations can be of practical value if they improve the prediction of the criterion variable for the subjects studied in the research, and if the predictions are equally good when the study is replicated with another sample of subjects. Where the purpose is to get the best possible prediction of a criterion variable, multiple correlations can be very useful.

MULTIPLE REGRESSION

Multiple correlation improves predictions by combining the predictive power of several variables. However, it does not provide information about the separate contribution of each variable. Several procedures based on multiple correlation do provide such information. They are called *multiple regression* techniques. If used and interpreted with suitable caution, they have a great deal of potential value for problems where group designs are inappropriate.

There are three main types of multiple regression. *Standard multiple regression* determines how much of the relationship between a set of predictor variables and a criterion variable is uniquely contributed by each of the predictor variables. For example, how much do each of the predictor variables of age and amount of hearing impairment contribute uniquely to the prediction of the amount of improvement with speechreading training? Such information could be very useful in assignments to groups for speechreading training, and in planning the total amount of training required for all groups.

A second type of multiple regression is *hierarchical regression*, where the amount that a new predictor variable contributes to a multiple correlation is determined. For example, researchers might want to know if a speechreading aptitude test score would add substantially to the prediction of improvement with speechreading training. The multiple correlation of age and hearing loss with amount of improvement would be determined, and then the amount of change in the multiple correlation after the aptitude test score was added as a third predictor variable would be determined. This procedure would be of practical use in determining whether the time and expense involved in estimating aptitude would be of sufficient predictive value in planning training programs.

The third type of multiple regression is *stepwise regression*. For a given set of predictor variables, what is the order in which to enter predictor variables into the multiple regression equation for the best prediction of the criterion variable? This is another way to select the best set of predictor variables, and to discard variables that do not contribute to the prediction.

Great care must be taken in using and interpreting multiple regression analyses. How much a given predictor variable contributes depends on its correlation with the other predictor variables. Preliminary research is helpful in selecting a useful set of predictors. Once the amount of predictive value of individual variables has been determined for one sample, a *replication* or *cross-validation* study should be carried out to determine whether the same results will be obtained with another sample. The ideal minimum number of subjects is 20 per predictor variable, and 10 subjects per variable is the practical minimum. The smaller the number of subjects, the greater will be the probability of overestimating the prediction. The need for large groups and for cross-validation is greatest for stepwise regression.

FACTOR ANALYSIS

Where measures of a large number of variables have been obtained for a group of subjects, they may be grouped into subsets of highly correlated variables called *factors* by factor analysis. First, the intercorrelations among all the measures are calculated, and then the intercorrelations are mathematically "rotated" to group the most highly correlated measures into factors. Several different methods of factor analysis are available.

Factor analysis may be used to reduce the number of variables to be used in further data analyses. For example, a number of language tests had been administered to a group of subjects who are language disordered and three factors had been found by factor analysis. The first factor included tests of word knowledge, the second, tests of syntactic knowledge, and the third, tests of discourse knowledge. For further research, the researchers could select the test that had the highest *factor loading*, that is, was most highly correlated with each factor. This would reduce the number of tests in the language test battery. Another procedure for reducing the number of variables in further research would be to use the *factor score* that is calculated for each factor as a composite score that best represents each factor. However, all of the original tests would have to be given to obtain the factor scores.

Great care must be taken in using and interpreting factor analysis. Factors are abstract entities, and should not be interpreted as actual abilities. The factors obtained depend on the variables included and on the characteristics of the sample of subjects. Preliminary research is recommended to select measures, and cross-validation is recommended to confirm the findings with another sample. A major obstacle is the requirement for large samples of subjects. Factor analyses usually involve at least 10 variables, which would require minimum samples of 100 to 200 subjects.

Q FACTOR ANALYSIS AND CLUSTER ANALYSIS

The most common type of factor analysis, called R *factor analysis*, as described previously, groups variables into factors on the basis of the intercorrelations among the variables for a group of subjects. Q *factor analysis* groups subjects rather than tests into factors. The subjects are grouped into factors on the basis of similar patterns of test scores. If several tests of different language abilities were given to children who are language disordered, and a Q factor analysis was carried out, one factor might include subjects with especially low scores on language comprehension and another factor might include subjects with low scores on language expression. With this technique, then, subjects might be classified into subtypes of HCDs.

Cluster analysis also groups subjects into subgroups on the basis of similar patterns of scores, but using a different statistical technique. There are a number of different methods for cluster analysis, and it is important to determine which is most appropriate for a particular problem.

Q factor analysis and cluster analysis are promising methods for identifying different types of HCDs. They use a different approach from group designs to determine the characteristics of HCDs. Instead of assigning subjects to groups and then determining their characteristics, Q factor analysis and cluster analysis begin with an unselected group of subjects and statistically classify them into subgroups with similar characteristics. However, the usual cautions apply to the interpretation of these analyses. The factors and the clusters are abstract entities, not actual subtypes of disorders. The factors and clusters that are found depend on the variables assessed and the characteristics of the samples of subjects, as well as the particular statistical technique used. Within each factor or cluster there may be considerable variability in the profiles of subjects.

ANALYSIS OF COVARIANCE

When a variable such as age needs to be controlled in a standard group design, the groups can be matched in age, or age can be systematically varied as one of the independent variables. Where the variable cannot be controlled in this manner, a statistical control procedure called *analysis of covariance* or ANCOVA can be used. The groups being compared are equated for the uncontrolled variable by a technique that adjusts the means in a manner similar to partial correlation.

ANCOVA can serve three purposes: it can increase the power of the statistical tests of the effects of independent variables by removing the within-group variance attributable to the uncontrolled variable, it can statistically match the groups for the uncontrolled variable, and it can isolate the effects of multiple dependent variables in multivariate analysis of variance. ANCOVA can be a very useful tool for HCD research when relevant variables cannot be controlled, as it permits valid group comparisons and increases statistical power. However, the adjusted means must be interpreted with caution, in the same way as partial correlations.

MULTIVARIATE ANALYSIS OF VARIANCE

In some research it may be of interest to have more than one dependent variable. For example, in studying the effects of therapy for voice disorders, researchers may wish to use both listener judgments and acoustic measures of voice quality before and after treatment. Both dependent variables can be analyzed by a single statistical procedure called *multivariate analysis of variance* or MANOVA. The two or more dependent variables are combined in such a way that they maximize differences between means for the main effects and interactions.

MANOVA serves several purposes. Error terms are chosen to adjust for the increased probability of chance differences with two or more dependent variables. The multivariate measure of combined dependent variables may provide a more sensitive test of the effects of the independent variable than would the separate dependent variables. Then the effects of the independent variables on each of the dependent variables separately can be determined by a procedure called *stepdown analysis*, where the dependent variables are tested in a series of ANCOVAs by a method similar to hierarchical analysis in multiple regression.

MANOVA can be useful in the early stages of research, where the researchers are not yet certain as to the most appropriate dependent variables to use for a particular problem. Where variables are uncontrolled, MANOVA can be combined with ANCOVA to produce MANCOVA, the most complex variation of ANOVA. Because of the increase of complexity and the possible difficulty of interpretation, however, researchers should try to select a single dependent variable that will be most sensitive to the effects of the independent variables.

DISCRIMINANT ANALYSIS

The final technique that combines group and correlational designs is *discriminant function analysis*, usually called *discriminant analysis*. The basic technique is identical with that for a simple MANOVA for independent groups. Two or more dependent variables are combined in such a way that they maximally discriminate between two or more groups. Discriminant analysis is usually used to discriminate natural groups. The dependent variables can be considered predictor variables and the group classifications criterion variables.

For example, researchers may wish to predict the occurrence of language disorders at age 4 on the basis of language and nonlanguage tests given to a sample of "at risk" two year olds. When the subjects have been classified into groups with and without language disorder on the basis of their language ability at age 4, a discriminant analysis determines the weighted combination of the scores of the tests given at age 2 that best discriminates the groups. Then a weighted score can be calculated for each child and the distributions of scores for the two groups can be compared to determine the amount of overlap in scores. If the dependent variables are not highly correlated, the group distributions may not overlap at all even though the distributions for each of the predictor variables do overlap. In such a case, the weighted scores for two year olds can be used to predict whether they will have a language disorder at age 4.

Discriminant analysis can be very useful for maximizing the accuracy of diagnosing HCDs. Like all other correlational procedures, however, discriminant analyses must be interpreted with caution, and no causal inferences can be made on the basis of discriminant analysis alone. There should be at least twice as many subjects in each group as there are dependent variables, with a minimum of 20 per group if at all possible. Where it is necessary to reduce the number of variables to accommodate small groups, multiple stepwise regression can be used to eliminate variables that contribute the least to the prediction. Cross-validation with another sample of subjects should be carried out to confirm the weighting of scores.

ADDITIONAL INFORMATION

Additional information about statistical analyses of correlations can be found in Edwards (1984) and Pedhazur and Kerlinger (1982) and other advanced statistics texts, with combined correlation and group designs discussed by Tabachnick and Fidell (1983) and other advanced statistics texts. There are also books devoted to specific techniques, including books on factor analysis by Cureton and D'Agostino (1983) and Gorsuch (1983), a book on cluster analysis by Lorr (1983), and books on multivariate analysis of variance by Barker and Barker (1984) and Bray and Maxwell (1985).

REVIEW QUESTIONS

1. Define the terms *covariance* and *regression*.
2. Give examples of high positive correlations and high negative correlations.
3. How are correlations used for predictions?
4. Create several sets of data involving 10 pairs of scores and make a scatter plot for each set. Try to make examples of high positive correlations, high negative correlations, and low correlations.
5. What information is obtained by squaring the correlation coefficient?
6. What are the effects of ceiling and floor effects on correlations?
7. How are correlations used to demonstrate reliability and validity?
8. What information is needed to calculate a partial correlation?
9. What is difference between partial and multiple correlation?
10. Describe the three types of multiple regression.
11. What is meant by factor loadings and factor scores?
12. How do Q factor analysis and cluster analysis differ from R factor analysis?
13. What are the three purposes for using ANCOVA?
14. What are the advantages and disadvantages of MANOVA?
15. What are the advantages and disadvantages of discriminant analysis?

CHAPTER

15

Analysis of Data Obtained with Other Designs

D ata analyses for standard group designs and correlation designs almost always involve statistics. Analysis of data for other research designs often involves other types of analysis.

OBSERVATION IN NATURAL SETTINGS

Both quantitative and qualitative data may be obtained from observations in natural settings. The data can be in the form of narrative records, field notes, or recorded units of behavior.

Narrative records are written descriptions of all details of the phenomena observed. The narrative can be used in its entirety to provide very detailed descriptive information, or can be abstracted and summarized for a more concise description. It can serve as a basis for qualitative analysis, or the observations can be coded into units of behavior for quantitative analysis.

Field notes are the selective verbal records of trained observers, as opposed to the complete descriptions contained in narrative records. The notes themselves can provide relevant descriptive information concerning the phenomena observed. They can serve as a basis for qualitative analysis, or can be coded into units of behavior for quantitative analysis.

Recorded units of behavior provide selective information concerning behaviors of interest, such as communicative interactions, that occur in natural settings. This information may be derived from narrative records or field notes, or may be obtained from direct observation of the events themselves or of audiotape or videotape records of the events. The units can be quantified in terms of relative frequency and duration, and there can be ratings of various aspects of the behaviors, such as a rating of emotionality of response on a seven-point scale. The quantified information can be further analyzed to provide descriptive statistics concerning averages and amount of variability. Statistical analysis of differences and relationships can also be carried out where enough subjects have been observed in particular types of situations.

Communicative Interactions

In HCD research, observation methods are used most often to study communicative interactions. In most cases, the basic data are units of communicative behavior such as demands, questions, requests for action, and comments. These data can be quantified in terms of relative frequency and duration, and can be rated on subjective dimensions. Sequential patterns of responses can also be quantified, such as the relative frequency of different responses to requests for action. Situational comparisons can also be made, such as the relative frequency of verbal and nonverbal communicative responses in the interaction of a child with HCD and a child without HCD as compared with the interaction of two children with HCD. Where appropriate, statistical analyses can be carried out to determine the significance of differences or relationships among communicative events.

CASE STUDIES

Case studies provide evidence about individuals that is not usually intended to be generalized to a population. Therefore, formal methods of statistical analysis are unnecessary. The data are quantitative and qualitative descriptions of a representative case of a particular HCD, a rare disorder, or a new treatment. Descriptions may be relatively brief or fairly detailed, sometimes book length. A great deal of the value of the case study depends on the researchers' ability to select and highlight relevant information, and integrate the information in a logical manner in relation to previous knowledge.

INDIVIDUAL DESCRIPTIONS

Individual descriptions of uniform physiological processes usually involve stable patterns of response, where statistical analysis is unnecessary. The descriptive data are directly interpreted. The data can be numerical quantities, verbal descriptions, and pictorial representations, and descriptive statistics may be presented in the form of tables and graphs.

GROUP DESCRIPTIONS

Where group descriptions take the form of normative information (e.g., linguistic analyses of spontaneous speech samples or ear drum movement in response to pure tones), descriptive statistics such as frequency distributions, means, standard deviations, and ranges may be used to describe the findings, along with verbal descriptions. Where group descriptions are based on questionnaires and surveys, frequency distributions and other descriptive statistics may be reported. Cross-tabulations of relative frequency of data in different categories may also be reported, and such data may be analyzed statistically by techniques such as the chi-square.

SINGLE-SUBJECT RESEARCH DESIGNS

Single-subject designs are usually intended to control individual behavior carefully enough that no further analysis is needed after the numerical results are presented in tables or plotted in graphs. Graphic analysis is most commonly used. The number or rate of responses during baseline and training periods is plotted on graphs and interpretation is directly based on graphic results without further analysis.

For certain purposes, statistical analyses of the results of single-subject designs may be carried out. Where this is done, the design may be modified to make it more like a group design. Where standard single-subject designs are used, the only appropriate statistic may be the interrupted time-series analysis. Statistical analysis may be necessary where the graphical data do not provide a clear indication of changes in response.

QUASI-EXPERIMENTAL DESIGNS FOR RESEARCH IN NATURAL SETTINGS

The data obtained by quasi-experimental designs are statistically analyzed. The nonequivalent control group design compares two nonequivalent groups, one of which has received training. The groups are compared in terms of change from a first to a second measure, between which one of the groups has received treatment. The nonequivalence of the groups is statistically controlled by analysis of covariance. The groups are statistically equated for their pretraining scores, permitting a direct comparison of posttraining scores. Other variables for which the groups are not equivalent, such as age, may also be covaried.

For interrupted time-series designs, a statistical procedure called an *autoregressive integrated moving average* (ARIMA) is carried out to demonstrate that the only significant change in performance occurred after the time series had been interrupted by treatment. For combined nonequivalent control group and interrupted time-series designs, both ANCOVA and ARIMA could be used.

Passive observation designs for evaluating naturally occurring causal relationships are analyzed by a variety of correlational procedures where the correlations are interrelated as a function of their temporal sequence. Some of these analyses are facilitated by computer programs.

QUALITATIVE METHODS

By their nature, qualitative methods do not involve quantification of the data or statistical analysis. Data analysis involves more than simply a recording of new facts. Observational data in the form of direct observations, videotapes, audiotapes, verbal descriptions, or verbal transcriptions may be analyzed, as well as other forms of data such as interviews, diaries, and personal reflections. Data collection, analysis, and interpretation may be merged in an ongoing process that leads to conclusions concerning the characteristics and the interrelationships of the processes of interest to the researchers.

The objective of qualitative analysis is to discover structure or meaning, not to make quantitative probability statements. Analysis and interpretation usually take place through several stages. The first stage may be a detailed description of the phenomena studied. This information can provide useful knowledge by itself. The second stage of analysis may involve interpretation with respect to the purposes of the research and to the interrelationships of the phenomena described in the first stage. In a final stage, the interpretations may be related to data from other studies and integrated into a theoretical explanation. There is an attempt to integrate results into an overall body of knowledge. As Chapter 16 will indicate, these stages of qualitative data analysis and interpretation are essentially the same as the stages of interpretation of quantitative data analyses. Both qualitative and quantitative methods arrive at the same end point, but by different routes.

There are a number of qualitative methods, and each analyzes data in a somewhat different way. There has been very little published HCD research using qualitative methods, but they may be very useful for investigating certain problems concerning HCDs. Some examples of qualitative methods of data analysis and interpretation will be given here.

Ethnographic methods are used to analyze observational data to determine the "native point of view" (Marcus & Fischer, 1986). Participant observers suspend their own point of view by "defamiliarization," and may then obtain insights regarding their own culture by "cross-cultural juxtaposition." Such methods could be used to study the effect of hearing impairment on communicative interactions in different cultures.

Phenomenological methods use descriptions of experiences. The researcher attempts to determine the essential structure of the phenomenon described by "empathic intuition" and a "bracketing" of prejudices and presuppositions. This shifts the focus from the objective to the experienced situation. In the analysis and interpretation, the researchers attempt to describe, understand, and finally interrelate the central themes. The goal is to discover the psychological structure of the phenomena studied. Such a method could be used to determine the existential-phenomenological experience associated with stuttering or with an acquired sensorineural hearing loss.

Hermeneutic methods interpret qualitative data by an analytic procedure called the "hermeneutic circle." The researchers begin with "pre-understanding" or presuppositions and then interrogate the confused and unclear "text," that is, observations. Then they reflect upon the pre-understanding in relation to the interpretation to come to a new understanding of the text. Such a method could be used to interpret the communicative intentions of persons with HCDs on the basis of their observed communicative interactions.

There are other qualitative methods in various stages of development. Some may be of particular use in HCD research. For example, dialectical psychology emphasizes the importance of uniting the interactions that occur within individuals to those that occur between individuals. Such a method might permit HCD researchers to discover useful information about the structure of communicative interactions.

Although qualitative methods of data analysis cannot be described as systematically as quantitative methods, they promise more external validity. Phenomena are described as they exist rather than in terms of artificially defined variables. Such methods may provide useful alternatives for quantitative methods.

ADDITIONAL INFORMATION

Additional information about the analysis of other designs can be obtained from the references listed at the end of Chapter 8. Aanstoos (1987) has summarized a number of qualitative methods of data analysis.

REVIEW QUESTIONS

1. Briefly describe the types of quantitative and qualitative data analyses used for each of the designs other than qualitative methods.
2. In recent issues of JSHR and JSHD, look for examples of data analyses of designs other than standard group designs.
3. Discuss how qualitative analyses differ from quantitative analyses, and briefly describe ethnographic, phenomenological, and hermeneutic analyses.

CHAPTER
16

Interpretation of Research

Interpretation is the culmination of the research. After the data have been collected and analyzed, the researchers have to evaluate the findings. Where a study had very specific and very limited goals, the interpretation may involve a simple list of the findings. In most HCD research, however, different aspects of the research are examined to reach conclusions concerning the amount and type of new knowledge.

The exact manner of interpretation depends on the aspect of HCDs studied and the purpose. There may be as many as six stages of interpretation:

1. Have the findings accomplished the purpose?
2. What limitations are placed on the interpretation by the design, procedure, and method of analysis?
3. How does the new knowledge relate to previous knowledge concerning the problem?
4. Can practical applications be recommended?
5. What further research is needed?
6. What final conclusions can be drawn?

The first three stages are usually included, but not necessarily in the order given here. Sometimes the limitations of the findings are discussed before the findings are related to previous knowledge. When findings do not agree with previous knowledge, the previous knowledge may be cited first, and then the lack of agreement discussed in terms of limitations of the particular approach used in the present study. Recommendations for practical applications and suggestions for further research may or may not be offered, and there may not be a final conclusion. As is the case for other research events, HCD researchers tailor the interpretation to meet the needs of their research.

The stages of interpretation can be illustrated by the hypothetical study of the benefits of training in speechreading used as an example for the factorial ANOVA in Chapter 13.

ACCOMPLISHMENT OF THE ORIGINAL PURPOSE

The purpose states what the researchers wish to find. The statement may be in the form of questions, hypotheses derived from a theory, or predictions based on past knowledge. As a first step in the interpretation of findings, the researchers decide whether the purpose was accomplished. In the study of speechreading training, the purpose was to determine the benefits of training for younger and older persons with acquired sensorineural hearing loss. The purpose could have been stated as questions: Will speechreading continue to improve as more training is given? Will younger persons benefit more than older persons? or as predictions: There should be steady improvement with training, and younger persons should improve more.

Evaluation of the findings in relation to the purpose would reveal that there was steady improvement in speechreading with training, and that younger subjects improved more. The basic findings can be stated in a clear and simple manner. This initial interpretation does not go beyond the immediate findings. Further interpretations are made in the later stages.

LIMITATIONS IMPOSED BY THE DESIGN, PROCEDURE, AND ANALYSIS

The evaluation of results in terms of the inherent limitations of the research events is a crucial point in the research. The researchers have done their best to fill an important gap in knowledge, and must now decide just what they have found. Their interpretation is limited by their own research events. They cannot draw conclusions about independent variables that were not varied, dependent variables that were not measured, and populations of subjects that were not sampled. Their conclusions are also limited by the exact procedures and methods of data analysis that were used.

Before the researchers decide on their contribution to knowledge, the limitations imposed by the design, procedure, and analysis must be reviewed. What independent variables were identified for study? Were relevant variables adequately controlled? To what extent did the study have internal and external validity? Were the dependent variables measured in a reliable manner? How large and representative were the samples of subjects? Were the procedures adequately defined and properly carried out? What kind of information was yielded by the data analyses? The entire machinery of the study may be reexamined. In most HCD research, compromises must be made in the ideal requirements for design, procedure, and analysis because of practical considerations. The effects of these compromises are considered at this stage of interpretation.

In the study of training in speechreading, specific amounts of training of a particular type were given to particular samples of younger and older subjects. Their progress was assessed by a particular test of word recognition, and the findings were analyzed by a particular statistical technique. The study was a relatively simple comparison of three different amounts of training with two different groups. In interpreting the results, the researchers should confirm that relevant variables were controlled. If unmatched groups had been used, the advantage of younger subjects might have been attributable to the tendency for younger subjects to have more education and less hearing loss. Training conditions should have been the same for both groups, with enough preliminary instruction and practice that older subjects would not be penalized. There should have been some basis for estimating whether the word recognition task predicted speechreading ability in natural situations. The effects of the ceiling effect for the younger subjects after 16 hours of training should have been carefully considered. Conclusions concerning the benefits of training should have been applied only to the specific training procedure that was used. Other aspects of the design, procedure, and analysis that might have affected the findings, such as the reliability of judging spoken responses, should also have been examined.

The extent to which limitations must be discussed depends on the characteristics of the study. If age, sex, education, hearing loss, cultural background, type of training, and longer periods of training had been included as independent variables, and both performance on a word recognition test and evaluation in a natural setting as dependent variables, the interpretation would be less limited. In a relatively modest study like the one cited here, where there were only two independent variables, one dependent variable, and small groups, the researchers' interpretation would be limited to the suggestion that training of a particular type and duration might have more benefits for younger subjects.

Investigations of the same topic using other designs would be interpreted according to the type of design. Single-subject designs would obtain more definite but more limited information about training effects for individual subjects, and be interpreted by the special procedures that have been developed for single subject designs (cf. McReynolds & Kearns, 1983). Qualitative investigations would go deeper into the impact of training on communication in different situations, and be interpreted by the special methods of qualitative research (cf. Goetz & LeCompte, 1984). Surveys might assess the benefits of training through questionnaires, and be interpreted by the standards of survey research (cf. Fowler, 1984). For each approach, the limitations imposed by the design, procedure, and analysis would have to be considered.

RELATION TO PREVIOUS KNOWLEDGE

Previous knowledge is reviewed by researchers to determine how much is already known or guessed about a problem. After the research is carried out, they must decide whether their findings confirm, contradict, or add new information to previous theories and research.

A review of previous knowledge about the benefits of training in speechreading might have revealed more informed guesswork than knowledge gained through research. There might be scepticism about the benefits of formal training, especially training in the recognition of visual cues for isolated speech sounds. The small amount of previous research might suggest some benefits for formal training, but be generally inconclusive. Within such a framework of previous knowledge, the findings might confirm the benefits of training, and provide new information about the effects of age.

Where the findings add a small, definite amount of new information, comparisons with previous research can be brief and concise. Where the findings are more complex, a detailed comparison of the design, procedure, and analysis of the past and present research may be necessary. For the present example, a fairly narrow interpretation in relation to previous research might be sufficient. Previous findings concerning the benefits of training in speechreading are supported and extended. Research on the same topic using different approaches might be more controversial and require much more extensive interpretation in relation to previous knowledge.

PRACTICAL APPLICATIONS

The possibility of practical applications of research findings depends on how definite the findings are relative to the theories used by practitioners. Where practice is largely based on informed guesswork and there is no potential danger in applying findings, researchers may suggest the possible benefit of practical applications. This might occur when there was a valid and reliable demonstration that a new approach was superior to a practical approach largely based on guesswork.

Before making such suggestions, it is obviously important to review previous knowledge and specify the limitations imposed by the design, procedure, and analysis. In the present example, it might be suggested that practitioners who had not found a highly successful procedure for training speechreading could try some variation of the procedure used in the study. However, suitable cautions would be necessary regarding the small restricted samples of subjects, the limited subject and task variables assessed, the single type of training, the limited amount of training, the single dependent variable, and the ceiling effect that limited the data analysis.

Suggestions for practical applications vary widely with the types of HCDs and the aspects of HCDs studied. In the majority of research, suggestions are very cautious, and often accompanied by statements that further research is required for more definite recommendations. Knowledge about HCD research strategies is very helpful for practitioners who wish to evaluate suggestions for practical applications.

FURTHER RESEARCH

As a direct consequence of assessing the limitations of their findings, relating the findings to previous knowledge, and deciding on practical suggestions, researchers can suggest what further research might be needed. This is another crucial point in research. The researchers have done their best to formulate and carry out research on an important problem, and have realistically appraised their findings. They are in a very good position to make specific suggestions about the further research needed to obtain useful information about the problem. At this point in the interpretation, additional results such as descriptive statistics, data for individual subjects, and qualitative data of various kinds might be useful in suggesting the direction of further research.

In some cases, no further information may be needed regarding the specific topic of research. In others, the results might point to the need for further studies of the same type, using additional independent and dependent variables to add systematically to the information provided by the first study. Where the findings have been sufficiently inconclusive, a completely different research approach might be suggested. Where knowledge about a problem can only be provided by a series of studies, suggestions regarding further research are of the greatest importance.

In the study of speechreading training, if the limited findings were interpreted as suggesting the usefulness of training, and present knowledge was considered inadequate, a series of studies could be suggested. Samples of subjects of different ages, sexes, education, hearing loss, and cultural backgrounds could be selected. Different types of training could be designed. Larger amounts of training could be given. Results could be assessed with several different dependent variables, and with long-term follow-up. If there was a question of the usefulness of speechreading training, research could be designed to compare speechreading training with other rehabilitation strategies. Different types of research design such as qualitative methods might be suggested for such research. All of these suggestions would be made with the practical goals of HCD research in mind.

CONCLUSIONS

In drawing final conclusions, researchers can speculate in general terms about the implications of their findings and the current state of knowledge about the problem. Examination of research reports in JSHD and JSHR suggests that final conclusions may restate the main findings, recommend practical applications, or suggest further research. HCD researchers do not lose sight of their goals, and draw conclusions on the basis of a careful interpretation of what they have found in relation to past knowledge. If they feel confident of their findings, they present them as new knowledge, and if the findings seem suitable in relation to present practices, they make recommendations for practical applications. If knowledge is still incomplete, they suggest the types of further research that are needed. The concluding statement completes the contribution to knowledge for this particular research. If the researchers feel that the topic is important enough to pursue, they will plan and carry out more research.

INTERPRETATION OF OTHER DESIGNS

The stages of interpretation described previously apply most closely to standard group designs. The interpretation of other designs may be different. Individual and group descriptions may not require much interpretation. In case studies there is usually no data analysis, and the results may be interpreted as they are presented. With qualitative methods, the stages of interpretation may be carried out as part of the data analysis, as discussed in the previous chapter. Observational data that are quantitatively analyzed, single-subject designs, and quasi-experimental designs are usually interpreted in the same stages as standard group designs. In studies that use combinations of designs, the interpretation may be more elaborate.

ADDITIONAL INFORMATION

Most of the books on research methods cited in previous chapters discuss the interpretation of findings. Methods of interpretation may differ greatly according to the type of design. For example, qualitative research is interpreted quite differently than quantative research, and there are a number of different methods for interpreting qualitative research.

REVIEW QUESTIONS

1. List the five stages that may be included in the interpretation of HCD research, and briefly describe each.
2. For current issues of *JSHR* and *JSHD*, list the stages of interpretation that are included. Interpretations are found in sections headed *Discussion*, *Conclusions*, and *Results and Discussion*.

CHAPTER

17

Research Strategies

HCD research does not simply consist of carrying out a prescribed set of activities with a fixed set of research tools. Modifications and compromises are always needed to accommodate the practical problems of HCD research. The purpose, design, procedure, and method of analysis have to be adjusted and readjusted until all fit together into a study that will provide the desired information about the problem. There are many different kinds of HCD research problems. An approach that is suitable for one problem will not be appropriate for another. The flexible planning required for HCD research is better described as strategy than as method.

Researchers must be concerned with all aspects of the search for knowledge, from the evaluation of the problem to the smallest details of selecting and instructing subjects and recording their responses. These activities require strategies that go beyond the specific research events discussed in previous chapters. When first learning to do research, there is a natural tendency to become preoccupied with the unfamiliar technicalities of particular research designs, procedures, and data analysis. To carry out effective HCD research, however, it is necessary to adopt a broad perspective concerning choices among alternatives at each stage of research. Designs, procedures, and methods of analysis are just tools, not the sum and substance of research. HCD research is a practical enterprise aimed at ingeniously using available tools to achieve new knowledge about HCDs.

How can HCD researchers learn research strategies? It is not possible for researchers to learn all there is to know about each type of design, procedure, and analysis. In all aspects of HCD research there has to be a balance of rigor and expedience. Researchers need to become familiar with the available alternatives without becoming an expert in every method. The purpose of this book is to provide the necessary information. When planning each stage of research, it is helpful to know enough about the various methods to consider each alternative before reaching a decision. Then whatever additional information is required can be obtained by referring to specialized sources of information. Familiarity with each research event is necessary. For example, researchers who do not understand methods of data analysis can make serious mistakes both in designing and interpreting research. Researchers who are not familiar with strategies, methods, and techniques relevant to the problem may not accomplish much. Nor will researchers who have learned only one research approach and apply it to all problems.

Thoughtfulness is an essential component of HCD research strategy. Before reaching decisions about each research event and agreeing on the final integrated plan, researchers need to do as much careful, constructive thinking as possible. Equal thoughtfulness is required for interpreting the findings. The most important contribution to knowledge may be the realization of what is *not* known.

An essential aspect of research strategy is continuing sensitivity to the degree of uncertainty involved in research. Researchers can have no prior assurance that they will achieve new knowledge. When planning research, however, they should make the best possible use of what is already known about the phenomena under investigation. Where previous knowledge has decreased uncertainty, specific predictions may be possible. This would permit planned comparisons, thereby increasing the power of the research. Where there is less previous knowledge and more uncertainty, researchers may sacrifice analytic power in order to assess a wider range of possible effects.

In seeking the most appropriate approach to a particular problem, researchers face the prospect that a method with acceptable internal validity will not have external validity, or vice versa. In such cases, the researchers could decide to use more than one approach. Where alternative approaches are used, one approach may have more internal validity and the other more external validity. A common strategy in HCD research is to obtain both descriptive information and statistically analyzed information. Statistical analyses are interpreted to arrive at definite conclusions, and the descriptive information provides suggestions for further research. Descriptive information can include detailed quantitative data that are not statistically analyzed, as well as subjective observations of the researchers and introspective reports of the subjects.

A similar strategy is the use of alternative approaches to a particular problem. Some problems lend themselves to alternative approaches. For example, the problem of how to help persons with acquired sensorineural hearing loss can be approached from at least two different perspectives. Quantitatively oriented researchers might obtain information about the benefits of speechreading training by a series of studies that systematically vary age, sex, education, amount of hearing loss, type of training, duration of training, and other relevant variables. Qualitatively oriented researchers might instead begin by interviewing persons with acquired hearing loss, their families, their friends, and their fellow employees to assess the effects of hearing loss. They would obtain information about situational variables such as family support and the communicative demands of different settings, and personal variables such as motivation, success in self-management of problems, and risk-taking in communication. Both types of approach should provide more useful knowledge about the important problem of improving the communication of persons with hearing loss.

STRATEGIES USED FOR SPECIFIC RESEARCH EVENTS

In addition to the overall research strategies, it is necessary to approach each research event as a strategist, not an inflexible methodologist.

Problem

The choice of a problem involves knowledge about research, theory, and practice related to the problem, plus thoughtful insight into the aspects of the problem most worth investigating. To have the required depth of information about particular problems, the best strategy for most researchers is to not study too many different types of problems at the same time. As described in Chapter 3, there is a wide range of HCD research problems that require quite different approaches. Researchers who divide their efforts among too many different problems may tend to approach each problem in too superficial a manner.

The choice of problem will also be influenced by the researchers' general preferences regarding the type of phenomena studied. Dimensions of preference regarding different subject matter would include peripheral — central, receptive — expressive, physiological — behavioral, and assessment — intervention. It is probably best for researchers to pick problems that fit their interests. However, the problem should not be viewed as the only one of possible interest.

Purpose

Once a problem has been selected, research strategies play a crucial part in deciding on the specific purpose. The researchers must evaluate both the current state of knowledge about the problem and the available designs and procedures before deciding on the purpose. They may choose to pursue a small amount of definite knowledge or a greater depth of less definite knowledge. Small, definite steps are taken by stating specific purposes, or formulating specific hypotheses and predictions. Larger steps are taken to study more general aspects of the problem. The statement of purpose determines whether there will be carefully preplanned comparisons or open-ended searches.

Design

In the selection of research designs, the basic strategy is to be thoughtful and well informed. Researchers should not impulsively select what seems to be the one obvious best design. Awareness that there is rarely a perfect design dictates a thoughtful strategy.

A series of decisions must be made in choosing the research design. The first is the general approach, which can range from quantitative to qualitative. The choice of approach is determined in part by the general attitudes of the researchers. Those who prefer to be cautious, orderly, and analytic may choose a quantitative approach, whereas those who take a more open, holistic view may choose qualitative approaches. Among the orderly and analytic, those who wish to arrive at general conclusions about populations may choose standard group designs, and those who wish to draw rigorous conclusions about individuals may choose single-subject designs.

Whatever the design, it must not be viewed as the best or the only possible approach. Attempts to make a particular approach fit all problems will not advance knowledge as much as more flexible approaches to research design. The choice of design should be dictated by the problem and the purpose as well as the researchers' preferences.

Where a particular design has been chosen, the researchers should keep in mind its advantages and disadvantages, as discussed in Chapters 7 and 8. Standard group designs that permit inferences about cause and effect may not be feasible. The designs that can be used may provide information only about relationships between the variables studied. Conclusions will usually be reached about average group performance rather than individual performance, and measures of variables may be crude and have doubtful reliability and validity. Researchers who use single-subject designs should keep in mind the difficulties of generalizing from individual performance to populations and from rigidly controlled experimental operations to real-life situations. Those who use observational approaches and qualitative methods should keep in mind the difficulty of drawing general conclusions from uncontrolled observations and achieving agreement with other researchers concerning subjective observations. Whatever design is selected, the best strategy for researchers is to adopt a suitably cautious attitude.

Researchers who choose group research designs have an additional problem of deciding whether to get limited but definite information with simple group designs, or to attempt to meet the requirements of complex designs and interpret the complex data that are collected. Strategies for choosing group designs can best be developed by experience, always remembering the need for effective compromise. Those who choose qualitative designs have additional problems of using complex procedures for analyzing and interpreting their data as they are gathered, and avoiding observer bias while studying their own mental processes and those of the person observed. Researchers who interpret case studies should have the experience and the aptitude for putting together diverse information about individuals and relating it to relevant theoretical and practical knowledge.

Procedures

Strategies for selecting procedures involve thoughtfulness in balancing the need for valid and reliable procedures against the availability of subjects, tasks, equipment, facilities, and research personnel. Hasty choices dictated by expedience may greatly limit the interpretability of findings. Over-concern about reliability and validity may delay or prevent the research. A strategy adopted by some researchers in circumstances where the choice between these extremes is too difficult is to carry out methodological research aimed at demonstrating the validity and reliability of procedures that meet the requirements of practicality.

Data Analysis

There are no perfect techniques of data analysis. As is the case for research designs, each has its advantages and disadvantages. Researchers must be flexible, ingenious, and well informed in selecting methods of data analysis. Where statistical analyses are involved, the researchers can get supplementary information about the findings from descriptive statistics. The examination of group distributions is especially helpful for interpreting significant and nonsignificant differences, and individual results provide useful indications of the representativeness of group findings. Where data are observational, researchers should not hesitate to quantify information that might be helpful in interpreting the special types of analysis required by qualitative methods.

When statistical analyses are used, the researchers must make decisions regarding statistical analysis at the time the research is designed. Planned comparisons should be used wherever possible, and designs that require accepting the null hypothesis (see Chapter 11) should be avoided by the use of more complex designs involving multiple levels of interactions rather than simple comparisons. Researchers should know the standards for statistical analyses of the professional journals to which research reports will be submitted, and make certain that the data analyses meet these standards.

Interpretation

The essential strategy for interpretation is to accomplish an orderly set of goals. Researchers should refer the findings to the stated purpose and to previous research; remain aware of the limitations imposed by the design, procedure, and data analysis; offer cautious recommendations regarding practical applications; make creative suggestions for further research; and arrive at appropriate conclusions concerning the contribution to knowledge. Specific strategies are to thoughtfully and correctly interpret interactions; be cautious about statements concerning causal relationships, correlations, and acceptance of the null hypothesis; evaluate the adequacy of relevant controls; and make thoughtful comments concerning the generality of findings. The findings should be interpreted in such a way that other researchers have the necessary information and the encouragement to proceed further.

THE NEED FOR MULTIPLE PERSPECTIVES

HCD research strategists recognize the limitations imposed by theories, designs, procedures, and analyses. As a result of these limitations, the knowledge obtained by HCD research is provisional, subject to change as different theories, designs, procedures, and analyses are applied to research problems. The goal of HCD research is not to discover unchanging universal truths. Any research approach is welcome that might provide useful knowledge about HCDs.

Recent recommendations concerning human science research (cf. Polkinghorne, 1983) fit the practical goals of HCD research. Knowledge gained by research is provisional because it is unavoidably influenced by the theories, designs, procedures, and analyses used in research, as well as the values and expectations of the researchers. To overcome the limitations of a single perspective, multiple approaches to research problems are recommended. Multiple perspectives converge on the essential nature of the phenomena under investigation, increasing the likelihood of useful knowledge.

Not all problems of HCD research require multiple perspectives. However, this pluralistic approach to human sciences is eminently suited to the concept of research strategy presented in this book.

THE FUTURE

HCD research takes place in the context of changing knowledge, theories, research methods, technologies, professional practices, and cultures. Research strategies that are appropriate now may not be appropriate five years from now. An important aspect of research strategy is to make appropriate adjustments to change in the context in which research takes place. Researchers must keep up with new developments and be prepared to adjust their strategies. Some of the changes that may be expected will be described here.

New Knowledge

Generally accepted knowledge about HCDs seems to accumulate very slowly and to be mostly related to peripheral speech and hearing disorders. There is no indication of a sudden increase in accepted knowledge concerning disorders that involve central processes. It will probably be many years before there is accepted knowledge concerning all aspects of HCDs. The knowledge base from which research problems emerge may remain fairly stable, with the major gaps in knowledge diminishing slowly.

Changing Theories

Theories concerning some peripheral speech and hearing disorders are fairly well established, based more on accepted knowledge than guesswork. However, there are as yet no generally accepted theories of central disorders involving perception, cognition, and language. Theorists and researchers are very actively engaged in developing and investigating such theories. HCD researchers must be well informed concerning the current state of theory. Especially important at present are theories concerned with the extent to which central processes are automatic and encapsulated as opposed to consciously controlled and highly interactive (cf. Fodor, 1983; Rumelhart & McClelland, 1986). Theories related to developmental disorders are even less well established. Theorists and researchers are only beginning to formulate and investigate explanations of how inheritance and experience interact in the development of perception, cognition, and language. Such theories are essential to research on developmental disorders. Research strategies must be applied with an awareness of the current status of relevant theories.

Although accepted knowledge concerning HCDs does not appear to increase rapidly, new gaps in knowledge become apparent with increased interest in interactive communication as opposed to more peripheral speech and hearing mechanisms. Theoretical demands have steadily increased as practitioners and researchers have become concerned with successively higher-level language disorders, progressing from syntactic to semantic to pragmatic disorders. If research interests shift to even more subtle aspects of communication, such as dialogical interactions (cf. Friedman, 1984), theoretical demands will become even heavier. For the future, then, researchers will have to keep up with changes in theories of both the development and mature functioning of perception, cognition, and language, and also with increasingly complex theories of communicative interactions.

New Research Approaches

It has been repeatedly emphasized in the preceding chapters that no research methods are perfectly suited to the practical needs of HCD research. More appropriate methods would be very helpful. In planning research, there is always a tension between the desire to obtain objective information about HCDs and the desire for a deeper understanding of HCDs. Standard quantitative designs tend to produce objective but superficial information, and qualitative methods tend to produce deeper but less objectve information. In psychology and related disciplines from which HCD research methods are borrowed, there are renewed efforts to develop methods that reveal more about the nature of mental processes. The mental processes that concern HCD research are language processes, including communicative intentions and dialogic interactions. As new methods for studying these phenomena are developed, HCD research strategists will have to be even better informed concerning the available options in designing research.

New Procedures

The extent to which research increases our understanding of HCDs is limited by the validity and reliability of research procedures. This is a very important consideration for effective research strategies. Any improvement in procedures such as language tests and tests of central auditory disorders as a result of increased technical knowledge and improved theories will be of great help to HCD researchers.

Technological Change

The major technological changes that will affect HCD research involve computers. Progress in computer applications will continue to have a very widespread impact on HCD research and practice. Computer applications include aids to communication, training procedures, stimulus generation, response recording, and data analysis. Researchers must be aware of the impact of technological developments on all aspects of research.

Changes in Professional Practice

As theories and knowledge concerning communication processes evolve, professional practices change. Audiologists have become concerned with rehabilitation as well as assessment, and with central as well as peripheral disorders. Speech-language pathologists have become concerned with pragmatic disorders. Professionals who work with children who are hearing impaired continue to seek better methods for developing communicative skills. As practice changes, the gaps in knowledge studied by researchers change. Research and practice interact. New practices create new problems to be studied by researchers, and successful research can result in new practices.

Cultural Evolution

During the past century, communication has played an increasingly important part in the world's cultures. Forms and functions of communication will continue to change in a computerized world beset with political, economic, social, and ecological problems. HCD researchers and practitioners will become concerned with both broader and more subtle aspects of communication. As communication via computers becomes universal and computers begin to talk and listen, the distinction between written and spoken language will change and new kinds of HCDs (e.g., computer illiteracy) will emerge. HCD research and practice will be shaped by the changing communicative demands of twenty-first century cultures.

CONCLUSIONS

The discussion of research strategies creates a picture of researchers as thoughtful, resourceful, cautious, well informed, open minded, and conscientious. What may not have been emphasized enough is that researchers should also be efficient, persistent, idealistic, and able to complete what they have started. Such characteristics are also, of course, desirable for practitioners. Few researchers have all of these qualities in full measure, but they can serve as a model for successful research strategists. Research reported in JSHR, JSHD, and other professional journals suggests that most HCD researchers do have the qualities necessary for the successful employment of effective research strategies.

The importance of research strategies emphasizes the need for interaction between researchers, theorists, and practitioners. There should be the smallest possible gaps between research, theory, and practice. Researchers cannot insulate themselves from the realities of HCDs. They have to learn about real persons in natural settings. There is no simple way to accomplish this. Some researchers attempt to find out how the separate parts work while trying to remain aware of the broader context of HCDs. Others attempt to understand more about the total life situation of persons with HCDs by observing communicative interactions in natural settings. Both types of effort are aimed at obtaining useful knowledge for theorists and practitioners.

Research is a commitment to explore the unknown. Research strategies are employed with an awareness of our ignorance. All knowledge is subject to change, including knowledge about the problems, purposes, designs, procedures, analyses, and interpretations that constitute the events of HCD research. Research provides a difficult but rewarding opportunity to extend the frontiers of knowledge about human communication disorders.

ADDITIONAL INFORMATION

Additional information about research strategies for HCD research can be found in Hegde (1987), McReynolds and Kearns (1983), Shearer (1982), Silverman (1977), and Ventry and Schiavetti (1980).

Discussions of the need for multiple perspetives in human science research can be found in Brewer and Collins (1981), Fiske and Schweder (1986), and Polkinghorne (1983).

REVIEW QUESTIONS

1. Briefly describe the general research strategies discussed at the beginning of the chapter.
2. Briefly describe the strategies used for specific research events.
3. Why are multiple perspectives needed for HCD research?
4. In what ways may research strategies change in the future?

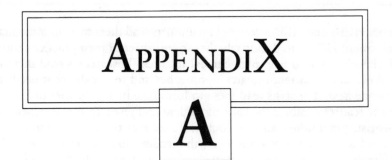

APPENDIX

A

How to Read and Evaluate HCD Research Reports

To be accepted for publication in an HCD journal, a research report must be carefully reviewed by two or three experts and found to meet the journal's standards regarding the quality of research and the style of presentation. The more familiar the reader is with the content and the style of research reports, the easier they are to read and to evaluate. Knowledge of the events that take place in research, as described in the preceding chapters, indicates what the contents of research reports will be. be. This appendix describes the style of HCD research reports, shows how to extract the information about research events from them, and gives guidelines for evaluating the research.

READING THE REPORT

Research reports must be carefully read in order to evaluate the findings of the researchers. Students read research reports to help them learn about HCDs and HCD research. Practitioners read them to learn something new about HCDs, to decide whether some aspect of their practice should be changed, and to help plan clinical research. Researchers read them to find out about current research approaches and to decide what needs to be done next. Theorists read them to formulate better theories of HCDs. Many readers combine the roles of student and researcher, researcher and theorist, practitioner and researcher. To extract the information that is needed for these various purposes, the reader must be familiar with the different parts of research reports and know how to find the different research events.

Research reports are most often published in professional journals. The leading American HCD journals are the *Journal of Speech and Hearing Research (JSHR)*, the *Journal of Speech and Hearing Disorders (JSHD)*, and the *Journal of the Acoustical Society of America (JASA)*. Most professionals read these journals to keep up with new developments in HCD research. As indicated in Chapter 3, there are a number of other journals concerned with HCD research, some general and some very specialized. All require that research reports be reviewed by experts before they are accepted for publication.

Research is also reported in other ways. Some projects are so large in scale that a whole book or monograph is needed. The research is reviewed by experts, but the style is less standard. Research reports are also published as chapters in books devoted to a particular topic. In such cases, there may not be a careful review, and the reports are often informal and incomplete. Before research reports are published, they are often distributed privately in the form of "preprints." Such reports have not yet been reviewed but are usually written in the style of journal articles. Research is also reported in unpublished theses which have been reviewed and approved by the candidate's thesis committee.

Parts of the Research Report

The research report is supposed to describe the background of the study and then state why it was done, what was done, what was found, and how the findings relate to previous knowledge, in that order. The information has to fit into the limited space available in journals and books, usually no more than 10 or 12 pages. If this cannot be done, the researcher must publish the report in monograph or book form or circulate a privately printed report.

Research reports vary in style from one journal to another and from one form of publication to another, but most include the following parts, which are listed in the order they occur in *JSHR* and *JSHD*:

- **TITLE**
- **AUTHORS**
- **ABSTRACT**
- **INTRODUCTION**
- **METHOD**
- **RESULTS**
- **DISCUSSION**
- **ACKNOWLEDGMENTS**
- **REFERENCES**
- **ADDRESS FOR REPRINTS**

To get an idea of what is included in each part, readers should look through the reports in an issue of *JSHR* or *JSHD* as each part is described here.

Title

The title may indicate something about the problem, the question, the research design, and the subjects. It may be possible to decide which papers to look at from the table of contents of a journal or book, or from a list of journal titles in a reference source such as *Current Contents*.

Authors

The authors are those who played a major part in finding the problem, planning the study, collecting, analyzing, and interpreting the data, and writing the report. The person who did the most is usually listed first, and may be the only author. Other authors may be members of a research team, or colleagues who gave special help with one or more parts. Where the institutional affiliation of the authors is given, it may provide some information about the context of the research.

Abstract

If the title does not give enough information, the abstract can be read for additional information. It summarizes the study in a few hundred words, with a sentence or two about the problem, question, design, subjects, method, results, and interpretation.

Introduction

The introduction begins the actual report, usually with no heading. It puts the research in context, establishes the necessity for doing it, and tells what is to be done. The authors begin by stating the problem and reviewing the most relevant theories, research, and practical implications. They usually specify the purpose and summarize the experimental plan, and may make formal predictions about the outcome. All of this is fitted into 1 to 3 pages. The review of previous research may be longer in cases where it is a new or complex topic, or shorter where the study directly extends previous research. Readers may have to peruse some of the reports of previous research cited in the *Introduction* in order to understand the present report.

Method

The *Method* section should give enough detail in 1 to 3 pages that someone else could replicate the study. It is usually divided into subsections with headings such as *Subjects*, *Materials*, *Procedure*, and *Data Analysis*, but HCD researchers often modify the headings to fit their study, as can be seen by looking through an issue of *JSHR* or *JSHD*.

The *Subjects* section is usually first, but sometimes the *Method* begins with an unheaded paragraph that describes the experimental design or a special technique used in the study. Such introductory paragraphs should be read carefully, because the authors have considered the material important enough to describe separately.

SUBJECTS. Almost all research reports have a *Subjects* section. This is especially necessary in HCD research, because the subjects are selected from special populations. The criteria for defining the HCD must be specified, and other information relevant to the study such as age, sex, intelligence level, socioeconomic status, and information about the HCD may also be given.

MATERIALS. Following the description of subjects, there is a description of the equipment, tests, or other materials used in the study. This section has headings such as *Materials*, *Apparatus*, *Instrumentation*, or *Tests*. The amount and type of details regarding materials depend on the study. It is important to determine the exact definitions of the independent and dependent variables. There may be reference to more complete information elsewhere. There should be enough information to permit replication.

PROCEDURE. After subjects and materials have been described, the procedure used to collect the experimental data is outlined. For studies involving training, the procedures used at each stage of training are outlined at some length. Where a single set of measurements is obtained in one testing session, the description of procedures can be shorter.

DATA ANALYSIS. In reports where the data analysis involves special techniques or is particularly complex, the analyses are described in a subsection in the *Methods* section. Otherwise they will be first mentioned in the *Results* section.

RELIABILITY. When the data are based on the judgments of observers, it is necessary to carry out special procedures to ensure that the judgments are reliable. These are often described in the *Methods* section.

Results

After the necessary information has been given about background, design, and experimental operations, the findings of the study are presented. In experiments where the results are not particularly complex, they may be combined with the interpretation in a section called *Results and Discussion*. The results are described in 1 to 4 pages, and may be divided into subsections that give the results for different groups, types of measurement procedure, or types of data analysis. The most important parts of the *Results* are often tables and graphs which present descriptive statistics and summarize the data analyses. These may be the essence of the findings.

Discussion

The results are interpreted in 1 to 3 pages in the *Discussion* section. The researchers return to the questions posed in the *Introduction* and decide how adequately they have answered them. Some authors stop there, but most try to relate the findings to those of previous researchers, discuss the practical and theoretical implications, and end with suggestions for further research. Some reports end with a subsection entitled *Summary* or *Conclusions* that summarizes the findings and interpretation.

Acknowledgments

Help given to authors is acknowledged in a footnote or a separate section. In *JSHR* and *JSHD* the acknowledgments follow the *Discussion*. In this section the authors acknowledge financial support by governmental agencies, private foundations, or others. They thank persons who gave advice about the research, made constructive criticisms of the written report, gave technical and clerical assistance, and provided subjects and testing or training facilities.

References

Published and unpublished books, journal articles, theses, and presentations at professional conferences referred to in the body of the paper are listed alphabetically in most journals in a standard format at the end of the research report. This section is essential. It gives information that may be needed to understand the background of the research report.

Appendices

Appendices are sometimes inserted after the references to provide more detailed information about materials or techniques.

Address for Reprints

JSHD, JSHR, and other journals give an address at the end of the paper (or in a footnote on the first page in some journals) where readers can send for a reprint of the paper. This may not be necessary, but it is very helpful for obtaining reprints of related research by the authors, especially research that has not yet been published. Most authors are generous in sending such information.

WHERE TO FIND RESEARCH EVENTS
IN A RESEARCH REPORT

Chapter 2 described the sequence of events in research and indicated where they could be found in research reports. There is not a perfect correspondence between the research events and the sections of research reports, but it is easy to find the events in the report. The problem is introduced at the beginning and the specific purpose is stated by the end of the *Introduction*. The design is often summarized at the end of the *Introduction* or at the beginning of the *Method* section. Further details of the design are often incorporated in the description of the procedure. The procedures are described in the *Method* section. The method of data analysis is described separately in the *Method* section or at the beginning of the *Results* section, or is described as the results are outlined in the *Results* section. Interpretations are presented in the *Discussion* section.

It may be helpful to go through an issue of *JSHR* and find the research events in each research report. The easiest to locate should be the problem, purpose, procedure, and interpretation. The details of the design and the data analysis may be spread over more than one section.

EVALUATING RESEARCH REPORTS

If publication in a journal, monograph, or book ensured that the research reported was perfect in all respects, the authors' interpretation could be accepted by researchers at face value. The findings could be added to the general knowledge, applied in practice, and used in designing further research. Perfection is rare in any type of research, and by its very nature HCD research tends to be less perfect than basic research into normal human processes. Basic researchers test abstract theories of normal processes with easily available normal subjects and carefully-controlled experimental techniques. HCD researchers confront the challenge of attempting to solve practical problems. They have to find representative subjects with HCDs, test or train them by whatever techniques are available, and control relevant variables as best they can. They cannot achieve perfection. It is important to evaluate their degree of success in order to decide how much their findings contribute to research, theory, and practice.

As described in Chapter 3, there is a wide variety of HCDs. The aspects studied and the techniques used are continuously changing. HCD researchers, like HCD practitioners, are necessarily self-taught in many respects. They do not usually work in a tidy, well-controlled laboratory. Their research reports reflect the pioneering nature of their enterprise. Those who evaluate research reports for professional journals and books are themselves self-taught researchers who volunteer their time for the difficult task of reviewing the research of others. Under these circumstances, it is encouraging that published research reports are as good as they are.

Because HCD research is so difficult, diverse, and changeable, why should anyone other than researchers even attempt to evaluate research reports? It is the best way to learn about HCD research. By carefully evaluating each research event readers can get a feeling for the challenge of HCD research. They can appreciate the usefulness of persisting in attempts to close important gaps in knowledge even though the theories, designs, procedures, and data analyses are not completely adequate for investigating the problem. If any published HCD study is carefully evaluated, shortcomings will be found. This is an inevitable result of attempting to answer practical questions.

General Strategies for Evaluating Research Reports

The evaluation of research reports requires an interesting type of research in itself. Like Sherlock Holmes, readers must search through the sections of the report to discover the researcher's motives and plans, and chart their actions. Then they become the judges who evaluate the evidence.

The first task is to find the research events described in Chapter 3. After evaluating each event, readers make an overall evaluation of the research report based on their knowledge of the topic. Research evaluation is a skill that is only acquired through practice. It requires background knowledge about research, theory, and practice. The critical attitude developed through evaluating research is essential for the professional who wants to meet the challenge of an ever-changing profession.

A potential stumbling block is lack of specialized knowledge about the problem and the usual methods of studying the problem. This can be avoided by only evaluating research reports within a particular field of interest. However, it is best not to completely restrict reading of research reports. Evaluating research reports on all aspects of HCDs is an excellent way for readers to broaden their knowledge about HCDs. This can be done by looking through all of the research reports in each issue of *JSHR* and *JSHD* (or other journals), and making a detailed evaluation of the research events in those papers that hold the most interest.

Readers should begin by seeing how much preliminary information can be obtained from the title and the abstract, and then work through the rest of the paper.

Evaluating the Problem, the Purpose, and the Design

The problem is always given in the first part of the *Introduction*, but it may not be divulged in full for a few paragraphs. The researchers should clearly relate the problem to a gap in knowledge about HCDs, but may not do so in studies concerning normal processes. There should be a description of accepted knowledge and theories concerning the problem, and a brief description of previous research directly related to the problem. If this information is not given, there is not an adequate basis for evaluating the contribution of the present study. Because of space limitations, readers may be referred to other publications for some of the essential information.

After the problem has been described, the purpose of the present research should be explicitly stated. This is done at the end of the *Introduction* in most research reports. When the purpose is stated, readers can evaluate the purpose to determine whether it seems sufficiently important and relevant to the problem. If the purpose is not specified, reader must review the rest of the report to infer what the purpose might have been. If the purpose cannot be determined, it will be difficult to judge the importance of the contribution to knowledge.

To evaluate the design, readers must discover where the essential details of the design have been described in the *Introduction* and *Method* sections. The design has to fit the purpose. Once the design is determined, readers can evaluate it to decide whether it will obtain the information about the problem specified by the purpose. Specialized knowledge about research designs, as given in Chapters 4 to 8, is required to evaluate the design.

Evaluating the Procedure

As described in Chapter 9, the exact operations for carrying out the design vary considerably from one research report to another. Care must be taken in evaluating each aspect of the procedure to make certain that independent and dependent variables have been adequately defined and relevant variables have been adequately controlled. This requires knowledge about theories, research methods, and practices relevant to the variables being investigated.

In evaluating subject selection, readers must determine how clearly the researchers defined the disorder, how representative the samples of subjects were of the total populations from which they were drawn, and whether groups of subjects were sufficiently matched on relevant variables. In evaluating assessment and training procedures, readers must decide whether the researchers have selected valid and reliable measures of the processes studied (see Chapters 4 and 9). In evaluating the remaining procedures, readers should decide whether all relevant situation variables have been controlled, or whether the lack of control of relevant variables will confound the interpretation of the findings. In particular, readers must determine whether the subjects were adequately instructed and motivated, and whether the effects of practice, fatigue, and boredom were avoided.

Evaluating the Data Analysis

Evaluation of the data analysis depends on whether the study involves a standard design with statistical analysis, a descriptive study, or a qualitative study using special procedures for data analysis. Where the data have been statistically analyzed, it must be determined whether appropriate statistical techniques have been correctly employed (see Chapters 10 to 15). Where descriptive data are used in observational, case history, and single-subject designs it must be determined that sufficient information is presented in appropriate form. Where qualitative methods are used, it must be determined that appropriate methods of analysis have been used (see Chapter 15).

Evaluating the Interpretation

Evaluation of the problem and the purpose requires judgments of the potential importance of the research, and evaluation of the design, procedure, and analysis requires judgment of the technical aspects of the research. The most crucial evaluation is of the interpretation, where the value of the study is decided by examination of the findings. It is first necessary to determine whether the researchers interpret the findings in relation to the purpose of the study, then the validity of the interpretation must be judged.

In research involving statistical analyses, a knowledge of statistics is necessary to determine whether the inferences concerning the statistical analyses are valid (see Chapters 10 to 14). It is not uncommon for researchers to conclude that the independent variables had significant effects when the statistical analyses do not permit such conclusions. It is even more common for the researchers to incorrectly conclude that a lack of a significant difference proves that there is no effect of an independent variable (see the discussion on accepting the null hypothesis in Chapter 11). The validity of the interpretation of studies that do not involve statistical analyses depends on the type of design and the accepted procedures for data analysis (see Chapters 8 and 15).

Most researchers are cautious in suggesting practical applications of the findings. When such suggestions are made, readers have to decide whether this interpretation is really warranted. If the measures are not sufficiently direct, or the sample of subjects not sufficiently representative, or the results of the analyses not sufficiently definitive, suggested applications may be dangerously misleading. Where there are suggestions for further research, readers might decide that other types of further research might have even more value.

By the time the researchers present final conclusions at the end of the paper, readers should be prepared to reach final conclusions regarding the contribution of the research, and to decide whether their conclusions agree with those of the researchers.

Final Suggestions Regarding Evaluation

Once the basic skills for evaluating the research have been developed, it is important to remember that all HCD researchers are doing the best they can with the tools at hand. Even when a study contains many imperfections, it may represent an effective strategy for obtaining as much of the desired information as possible. Not only must each research event be evaluated separately, but the total strategy of the researchers must be evaluated at the time of reaching a final conclusion concerning the contribution to knowledge (see Chapter 17).

Familiarity with the events of HCD research, as described in the preceding chapters, provides a necessary perspective for evaluating research. Skills for evaluating published research are built up by regularly reading published research with an informed critical attitude.

ADDITIONAL INFORMATION

Light and Pillemer (1984) devoted an entire book to the science of reviewing research. Other suggestions for evaluating different aspects can be found in the references given at the ends of the preceding chapters.

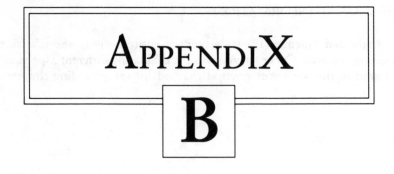

APPENDIX

B

How to Plan, Carry Out, and Interpret HCD Research

A ll of the information given in the preceding chapters and in Appendix A is useful for planning, carrying out, and interpreting research. The more familiar researchers are with research methods that may be appropriate for the problem, the better the research will be.

THE REASONS FOR DOING RESEARCH

The reasons for doing the research are important. If the research is a student project, it cannot be too large a study in terms of design, procedure, data reduction, or data analysis. It may not be possible to meet all of the requirements for design and data analysis. Student projects should be restricted in scope, perhaps to simple group designs or case studies, and can be presented as exercises or preliminary studies.

For student theses, the research should be much more substantial. The research must meet the standards set for the thesis examination process, and should usually involve generally accepted approaches to a problem. Where a student wishes to use an innovative approach, there should be careful consultation with the supervisor.

To learn how to do research, students doing projects or theses should make their own decisions concerning all aspects of the research whenever possible, and try to become experts on the topic. Students who rely on supervisors, statisticians, and others for decisions are not likely to become researchers who contribute important new information about HCDs.

For research that will be submitted for publication in research journals, the standards of the journals should be determined regarding numbers of subjects, types of designs, and data analyses. Where there are too few subjects, flaws in the design, or inappropriate data analyses, there will be difficulty publishing the findings in a leading journal.

For research plans that will be submitted to government agencies, private foundations, or other sources to obtain funds needed for the research, it is very important to meet the standards set by the funding agency. The standards may vary considerably from one agency to another. Government agencies usually set very precise criteria for the importance of the problem, the thoroughness of the review of relevant literature, the number and type of subjects, the appropriateness of the design and data analysis, and the approval of an ethics committee. Private foundations may use less strict criteria, but may support a more restricted type of research. Researchers should familiarize themselves with the exact research criteria and with the exact type of research funded before writing proposals for funding. A great deal of time and effort may be expended for nothing if researchers do not pay sufficient attention to these important details.

Where the research is based on previous investigations by the present researchers or others, all of the details of the previous research should be reviewed. This should be done in as critical a manner as possible. There may be relevant research, theories, or practical issues that were not considered, perhaps because they involve new information. Improvements in the designs or analyses may be possible, or alternative approaches may provide fresh perspectives. Where there is sufficient information about a problem from past research, the researchers have to plan research that will provide an important confirmation or a significant extension of the previous findings.

Where preliminary or exploratory research is undertaken, researchers should use their imagination, ingenuity, and previous knowledge to the fullest. The first study on a problem should be broad enough in scope to suggest the most promising directions for further research.

TYPE OF RESEARCH

Another important consideration when beginning to plan research is the type of research. This will depend on both the interests and inclinations of the researchers. Researchers usually restrict their interests to one field (e.g., audiology, education of children who hearing impaired, or speech-language pathology), to one type of disorder within the field (e.g., peripheral auditory disorders or speech disorders), and, in some cases, to one aspect of one disorder (e.g., lip movements in stutterers). To the extent that there is accepted knowledge as opposed to guesswork concerning the disorders studied, research planning can be solidly based on previous knowledge. Research based on broader aspects of communication will tend to have a less definite knowledge base. Some researchers may prefer to work on more definite problems, and others on problems where the frontiers of knowledge are uncharted.

RESEARCH APPROACH

Once the type of research is selected, researchers have to decide on the type of approach. In most cases, approaches used by previous researchers for similar problems will be selected. Quantitative approaches using standard designs and statistical analyses are selected for most HCD problems. However, for problems involving broader aspects of communication, qualitative approaches using innovative methods may be selected. There is a tendency for researchers studying peripheral processes to use quantitative, analytic approaches, and for researchers studying more central processes to use qualitative, holistic approaches (see Chapter 17). There is also a tendency for the use of quantitative approaches for research concerning assessment, even where more central processes such as syntactic abilities are involved. Both quantitative and qualitative approaches are used for research concerning intervention.

Researchers must decide whether to use group designs or individual subject designs. Group designs are still most common in *JSHR* and *JSHD*, but other designs are often useful. Case studies may be used in the early stages of research on a problem. Single-subject designs may be used where the researchers have definite hypotheses about an effective form of intervention. Observational methods seem most appropriate at the present time for studying communicative interactions of small numbers of subjects.

The choice of approach not only depends on the type of problem, but on the potential advantages and disadvantages of each approach. Quantitative approaches tend to yield definite but limited knowledge. Qualitative approaches tend to yield unlimited but indefinite information. Studies of individuals provide detailed and definite information, but are difficult to generalize. Researchers who are seriously concerned with the choice of approach can find many lengthy arguments for and against each type of approach (see Chapter 17). However, HCD researchers tend to be more concerned with the achievement of useful knowledge than with the exact approach used.

COLLABORATIVE RESEARCH

Research may be carried out by pairs of students, a student and supervisor, a student and thesis committee, pairs of researchers, teams of researchers, or one solitary researcher. Chance plays a part in the effectiveness of each form of collaboration. Different persons have different talents. Some are best at suggesting ideas for research, and others at searching the literature, making effective designs, planning and carrying out procedures, analyzing data, or interpreting the results. Collaboration can be useful for arriving at common decisions at each stage of research, or for allowing collaborators to be responsible for the parts that suit their talents. Those who want to be able to function as independent, self-sufficient researchers should participate in all aspects of research.

GENERAL STRATEGY

Thoughtfulness is essential for each stage of planning, carrying out, and interpreting research. Research requires a large intellectual and emotional investment. Every effort should be made to avoid hasty decisions, easy solutions, and convenient shortcuts. Poorly conceived, executed, and interpreted research is embarrassing for everyone concerned, and will not increase knowledge about HCDs.

Researchers have to proceed in a thoughtful, responsible manner with the realization that they cannot know everything about the problem, research designs, procedures, and methods of data analysis. They must learn as much as they can and then do the best they can. Those who find HCD research a formidable prospect should begin by choosing definite problems that can be studied by orderly methods.

The potential rewards for researchers are great. Some of the most important advances in science are made by clever students who bring a fresh perspective to a problem. Appropriate training and hard work are necessary elements. Chance plays an unavoidable role, or else research would not be research. The final ingredient is thoughtfulness.

HOW TO START

If researchers do not have a pressing problem that demands investigation, there are several ways of finding one. Obvious approaches are to read relevant literature concerning research, theory, and practice, and to consult other researchers, theorists, and practitioners. Another strategy is to keep a list of problems as they come to mind, and then get the opinions of others concerning their potential importance. Some problems that seem very important at first do not stand up to later scrutiny.

Once a potential problem or problems have emerged, possible approaches can be considered. Is it a large problem that requires extensive planning, a smaller study that can be carried out with limited resources, or a new idea that requires preliminary exploration? This is a stage where time must be set aside for thoughtful reflection as opposed to impulsive decision making, or the researchers may find themselves launched on an unsuccessful enterprise. Advice may be sought at this stage from those who use different approaches.

At some point, a decision is made to proceed further with the problem. Then the research is underway, at least in a preliminary manner, and the next stages of planning can proceed.

REVIEW OF THE LITERATURE

After a possible problem has been selected, the exact purpose of research on the problem cannot be determined without a thorough search of the literature. The best strategy is to find the most recent publications concerning the problem, particularly reviews of research and theory. This can be done by reading current issues and annual indexes of *JSHR* and *JSHD* and other appropriate journals, looking through reference sources such as *Current Contents*, writing to researchers who have studied the problem, and using bibliographic search procedures such as *Medline* and *Science Citation Index*. As information is gathered, the current status of both theories and research should be carefully evaluated (see Appendix A) to define an important gap in knowledge concerning the problem.

PLANNING THE RESEARCH

When the literature has been reviewed, the purpose can be defined in relation to an important gap in knowledge. Then further planning of the design, procedure, and analysis can proceed. If the original purpose cannot be carried out because of limitations imposed by the design, procedure, or analysis, it is modified accordingly.

Once a tentative purpose has been defined, there is a temptation to select an obvious design. It is best to take the time to consider a variety of designs before reaching a final decision. This is where a team of researchers and consultants with different experience and viewpoints regarding research designs can be helpful. An essential aspect of this phase of planning is the identification of independent variables, dependent variables, and relevant variables that must be controlled.

When a design has been tentatively selected, the researchers must determine whether an acceptable procedure can be formulated. The first considerations are whether subjects are available in sufficient numbers, and whether relevant variables can be defined and controlled. Where the variables to be studied are not well defined, it may may be difficult to decide on valid and reliable procedures for assessing or manipulating the variables. Needs for equipment, facilities, and technical assistance must be carefully considered to determine whether available resources are sufficient. If not, assistance must be sought from outside sources.

Where qualitative methods and single-subject designs are used, data analyses may be planned as the data are being collected. Where quantitative group designs are used, methods of data analysis should be decided upon before final decisions are reached concerning the purpose, design, and procedure. Such forethought seems to go against human nature. Even experienced researchers may not explicitly plan the data analysis until the data have been collected. However, there are two important dangers in not planning the data analysis ahead of time. First, the choice of analyses may be biased by prior examination of the data. Such bias makes the probability estimates obtained by statistical analysis meaningless, and invalidates the contribution to knowledge about HCDs. Second, if the data analysis methods are not selected in advance, the researchers may find that their data do not meet the requirements of the available methods of analysis. In such a case, the data will be uninterpretable and will not contribute to knowledge about HCDs. In addition to avoiding these dangers, planning the data analysis at the time of designing the study can have an important advantage. Researchers may be able to make planned comparisons on the basis of previous knowledge and theories, and thus increase the chances of a contribution to knowledge about HCDs.

Once the best possible adjustments of the plan have been made to integrate the purpose, design, procedure, and analysis, a final plan can be decided upon. At this point, the researchers should take the time to review the plan to determine whether there have been any oversights, or whether any alternative approaches have suggested themselves. The final outcome of the research should be carefully considered. In adjusting their plans for the separate parts, researchers may lose sight of how their findings are intended to contribute useful knowledge about HCDs.

PRELIMINARY STUDIES

If there has been little or no previous research on a problem, the researchers may not be able to tell in advance whether their plan will result in useable data. For example, if an experimental task has not been used before with subjects with HCDs, the researchers may not be certain that the subjects will understand the task. The task may be too difficult for HCD subjects, resulting in floor effects, or too easy for control subjects, resulting in ceiling effects. In such cases, a small preliminary study can be very helpful in planning the exact procedures that will be used. Pilot studies are also helpful when researchers are applying for funds for research on a new topic for which previous research cannot be cited. Granting agencies are never as optimistic as the researchers themselves about the chances of a contribution to knowledge.

DATA COLLECTION

When the final plan is put into action, the data are collected. Data collection must take place exactly as planned. Otherwise, the data may be meaningless or misleading. The data have to be collected in a careful manner, and researchers must ensure that those who gather the data are reliable and conscientious, especially where the data are gathered in an unsupervised situation. The researchers must have a responsible attitude toward their research. Anyone who collects data in a careless manner may harm themselves, their profession, and persons with HCDs.

DATA ANALYSIS

Where data analyses have been planned, they must be carried out according to plan. Great care should be taken to calculate and display descriptive statistics that reveal the salient features of the data. Such displays can take the forms of graphs or tables. Great care should also be taken in presenting the results of complex analyses such as higher-order interactions (Chapter 13) and multivariate correlation analyses (Chapter 14).

Where data are qualitatively analyzed, the analysis may take place as part of the data collection, and should proceed according to the established conventions of the qualitative method used (Chapter 15).

INTERPRETATION

The researchers' job is not finished when the data have been collected. It is their responsibility to determine the extent to which the purpose has been achieved, to relate the findings to previous research, and to describe the contribution to knowledge. Whereas the previous research events have required a great deal of deductive reasoning, the interpretation requires inductive reasoning. The researchers must determine the implications of the findings as well as understand the findings themselves. Then the interpretation can be extended to suitably cautious recommendations regarding practical applications, and useful suggestions can be made regarding the most promising directions for further research (Chapter 16).

Where the researchers have found an important problem and given their most thoughtful attention to each phase of planning, data collection, and data analysis, the interpretation is the culmination of their work.

FUNDING

When an extensive research program is planned, or when a particular project involves unusual expenses (e.g., for equipment or travel), the researchers may have to obtain a relatively large amount of money in order to complete the research. This requires the preparation and submission of a research grant application. A great deal of time and effort is required to prepare applications. They have to be done in a certain form, and a great deal of information must be presented in a limited amount of space.

A potential drawback is that the chances of being funded may be small, especially where a nontraditional approach or a controversial topic is involved. Many researchers may hesitate to devote their time to a doubtful enterprise. Some researchers may lack the patience to follow the rigid formats of applications, and some may resent the idea that their choice of research is dictated by its potential acceptability to a funding agency.

These are important considerations, but there are also potential benefits in applying for funds. The researchers are forced to do thoughtful planning at each stage—to select an important problem, present a succinct literature review, define an explicit purpose, choose an appropriate design, attend to all details of procedure, and plan the data analysis. Having done this, they have the advantage of the peer review process. The application is reviewed by experts in their field, and the researchers are provided with the critical comments of the reviewers. This advice can be worth a great deal to the researchers in suggesting how the research plan could be improved. Then the researchers may be successful in further efforts to obtain funds.

ETHICAL CONSIDERATIONS

Ethical considerations in HCD research relate to the researchers' responsibility to plan, carry out, and report the findings of research in a responsible manner, and to deal with subjects in an ethical manner. The institutions that employ researchers and the agencies that grant them funds require all research proposals to be reviewed by an ethics committee to guarantee the use of ethical procedures. These include not exposing subjects to physical or psychological risks, obtaining informed consent from subjects (and, where necessary, parents and teachers), not deceiving subjects regarding the purpose of the research, and not divulging private information about the subjects. Standard forms are required for obtaining the informed consent of subjects and for certifying the approval of an ethics committee. Researchers have to be aware of ethical considerations in planning research, and take the necessary steps to ensure that ethical requirements have been met. Unethical practices with regard to the the treatment of subjects and to the research itself can have grave consequences for all concerned. Similar ethical considerations apply to animal research. A few unethical researchers can cast suspicion upon the whole research enterprise, and prevent the carrying out of research that might be of great benefit to persons with HCDs.

COMPLETING RESEARCH

After reading the preceding chapters, the preceding appendix, and this appendix, it should be obvious that a great deal of thought, study, and effort must go into any research, no matter how modest. Many different skills must be brought to bear before the research can be completed. The final product cannot be a perfunctory effort—it must be a useful contribution to knowledge. Unfortunately, many research projects are never brought to the final stage of completion. Like many other worthwhile enterprises, research requires sustained effort, a drive for completion, and a useful product. Anyone who does not feel equal to the challenge should think very seriously before undertaking research. For those who accept the challenge, the rewards can provide lifelong satisfaction, and can be of benefit to many future generations of persons with HCDs.

Research is not completed until it is available in published form. Appendix C describes this final phase of research.

ADDITIONAL INFORMATION

Most of the books cited in previous chapters on research methods in HCDs and in psychology contain suggestions about how to plan, carry out, and interpret research. Other books contain specific advice about student research (Smith, 1984), suggestions for reviewing the literature in planning research (Borchardt and Francis, 1984), and guidelines for obtaining funding (Quarles, 1986). Most books on research methods discuss the ethics of research. Very explicit guidelines are given in a publication entitled *Ethical principles in the conduct of research with student participants*, which can be obtained from the American Psychological Association, P.O. Box 12710, Hyattsville, Maryland 20784 ($8.50 plus $2.00 postage).

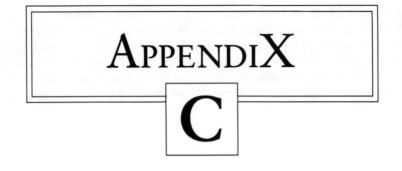

APPENDIX
C

How to Write Research Reports

T he final outcome of most research is a research report. It may take a number of different forms, such as oral presentations at seminars and professional meetings, theses, monographs, chapters, and books. The traditional form of contribution to knowledge is submission of a research report for publication in a professional journal. The report is reviewed by journal editors and expert consultants. If they recommend acceptance, the report is published and becomes a formal contribution to knowledge. They may also recommend revision and resubmission, or rejection. The care taken in planning, carrying out, and interpreting the research, as described in Appendix B, will largely determine the chances for acceptance and publication.

Suggestions for writing a research report for publication in a professional journal are given first, since the requirements for published reports are the most standard and rigorous. Then suggestions are given for other forms of report, including student projects, theses, and reports intended for oral presentation.

GENERAL WRITING STYLE

Several basic rules should be followed regarding the writing style for research reports:

1. Practice makes perfect. Writing style should improve with each research report, providing writers make a conscious effort to improve.

2. Researchers should revise everything they write. Most professional writers make endless revisions. Amateurs cannot expect to get it right the first, second, or even the third time.

3. Researchers should ask others (fellow students, supervisors, colleagues) to make comments and suggestions after they have completed a draft of the report. The most valuable suggestions may come from persons who have published a number of research reports themselves. They should be asked to be as critical as if they were reviewing the report for publication in a professional journal. This can be a great help in achieving an effective writing style.

4. Researchers should find a person who has written clear and concise research reports on the same general topic. They should use this person's writing as a model until they have developed their own effective style.

SPECIFIC WRITING STYLE

Each journal has its own style. Style requirements are usually given at the beginning or the end of each journal issue. For *JSHR* and *JSHD* there is a page at the end of each issue headed *Information for Authors*. Instructions are given regarding the type of research reports published in the journal, the procedure for reviewing reports submitted, the number of copies to be submitted, and the style to be used for tables, figures, and references. *JSHR* and *JSHD*, like many other journals, require that papers follow the style specified in the APA manual (*Publication Manual of the American Psychological Association*, 3rd edition, 1983). This manual gives specific instructions for preparing each part of the report, plus general suggestions about writing style, grammar, and other useful information. It is the best style manual of its type and is highly recommended for anyone who prepares research reports. The APA manual can be purchased from the American Psychological Association, P.O. Box 2710, Hyattsville, Maryland 20784 ($16.50 plus $2.00 postage).

Where there is any doubt concerning style, researchers should consult the journal to which the report is to be submitted. They should look through a current issue to find an example of the aspect of style in question. While writing the paper, it is best to find a similar report for use as a model in the journal to which the report will be submitted. The report should be of good quality in both content and style.

CONTENT

Suggestions regarding the content of research reports will refer to the guidelines of *JSHR* and *JSHD*. Some modifications will be required for other journals. These are easily determined by consulting a current issue of the journal. The kinds of material to be included in each section have been discussed in the previous chapters and appendices.

Title

The title briefly describes the research, usually in 15 words or less. It should be as brief as possible, and indicate the specific purpose of the research. Consult the title page of a current issue of *JSHR* or *JSHD*.

Authors

Authors are usually listed in the order of the importance of their contribution to the research. Research assistants and technicians who carried out instructions but did not contribute to decision making are usually not included. Researchers should see the APA manual for specific guidelines concerning authorship, and *JSHR* and *JSHD* for the listing of institutional affiliations.

Abstract

The report begins with an abstract of the study in 150 words or less. The abstract describes the problem, purpose, and design in about one sentence each, and the procedure, results, and discussion in one or two sentences each. Researchers are directed to the APA guidelines and specific examples in *JSHR* and *JSHD*.

Introduction

The introduction is the first section of the written report, and usually has no heading. Examination of an issue of *JSHR* or *JSHD* will reveal that the introductions may be very brief. They usually range from about 250 words (one double-spaced typewritten page) to 1,500 words (six double-spaced typewritten pages). As described in the preceding chapters and appendices, the introduction should succinctly describe research, theory, and practice relevant to the problem, the problem itself, and the specific purpose. The design is often summarized at the end of the introduction. Researchers are directed to the APA manual for general guidelines, and articles on similar topics in *JSHR* or *JSHD* for specific examples.

Method

The method section is usually relatively long, since it contains subsections describing the subjects, equipment, materials, and procedures. An introductory paragraph describing the design and a final subsection describing the data analysis may also be included. Enough details must be given for other researchers to repeat the study. Researchers should see the preceding chapters and appendices and the APA manual for general guidelines, and articles on similar topics in *JSHR* or *JSHD* on similar topics for specific examples.

Results

The results present the data gathered in the study, plus the results of data analyses. The writing of the results section is part of the research itself, since decisions regarding the final organization and presentation of the findings are often not made until the results section is written. General guidelines are given in the preceding chapters and appendices and the APA manual, and papers on similar topics in *JSHR* and *JSHD* should be consulted for specific examples. Authors should make every effort to present all the data that may be useful to readers. A great deal of care should be taken in deciding what data to include and in preparing tables and figures. Where sufficient information is given in the proper form, readers who are familiar with the research topic can often interpret the findings for themselves. As researchers become experienced in critically evaluating published research and in searching the literature for topics of interest, they will see the great value of clear and detailed presentation of results.

Discussion

The interpretation of results in the discussion section tends to be relatively long, and quite variable in both style and content. There may be a combined results and discussion section, a separate discussion section with or without subsections, or several final sections with specific headings such as *Considerations for Future Studies* and *Conclusions*. Even more than is the case for the results section, the writing of the discussion section is usually part of the research itself. The researchers often do not arrive at a final interpretation of their findings until they have to write the discussion section.

The style of the discussion section may vary from a very narrow operational description of the results to a lengthy, far-reaching interpretation. Usually, the main findings are summarized and related to the purpose at the beginning of the discussion. Then, limitations imposed by the design, procedure, and analysis are considered, and the findings are related to previous research and theory. Finally, recommendations may be made for practical applications and further research, and general conclusions stated (Chapter 16). General guidelines are given in the preceding chapters and appendices and in the APA manual, and specific examples of research on similar topics can be found in *JSHR* or *JSHD*.

The writing of the discussion should involve the most thought, the greatest care, and the most revisions. It sums up the writers' contribution to knowledge. As can be seen by reading research reports, sometimes the contribution is a small, specific increment of knowledge that can be briefly and succinctly described, sometimes the writers extensively interpret complex findings, and sometimes they use all of their eloquence to persuade readers of the importance of a new approach or a new topic. This section is usually the most difficult to write, but is the authors' opportunity to put the final touches to a lasting contribution to knowledge. The manner in which results are interpreted is an important factor in determining the impact of the report and the frequency with which the research is cited in subsequent reports.

Acknowledgment

In a brief section following the discussion, the writers should acknowledge help received from colleagues in planning and writing, from representatives of institutions in making subjects and facilities available, and from granting agencies for providing funds for the research. Guidelines are given in the APA manual and examples can be seen in *JSHR* and *JSHD*.

References

References must be cited in the text of the article in a standard manner, as dictated by the journal or book editors, and a list of references must be given after the acknowledgments, also in a standard manner. All references in the text and the reference list should be double- and triple-checked for exact accuracy. Incorrect references are very obvious to the experts that the writers of the paper most wish to impress.

Appendices

Details of tests and other technical information that might be of use to readers are presented in about 20 percent of the papers in *JSHR* and *JSHD* in appendices after the references. Guidelines are given in the APA manual and examples can be found in *JSHR* and *JSHD*.

OVERALL WRITING STRATEGIES

It is not necessary to write the sections of the research report in the order in which they appear. Where there are several authors, they may share the task and write the sections that suit their abilities and interests. Where there is a single author, the sections can be written as it suits the author's convenience. For beginning writers, the first step may be to assemble a folder of notes concerning each section. Whenever there is a pertinent thought or a specific detail that could be reported, it can be put on a piece of paper and stored in the folder. At some point, a draft of the section can be written on the basis of the notes. The draft should be revised several times until an acceptable first draft has been completed. In this manner, a complete draft can be assembled for comments and suggestions by research collaborators, fellow students, supervisors, or colleagues.

A convenient order of writing sections for beginning researchers may be to make a rough, perhaps overlong, draft of the introduction, and a more careful draft of the method section. Then a thoughtful draft of the results should be written. While this is being done, the writer should assemble notes for the discussion. When beginning the discussion, there may be a lack of interpretive ideas to add to the bare facts of the results. Prior notes can be very useful. It is also helpful to think about the interpretation whenever there is an opportunity for reflection. Often, the final stage of writing is completion of the introduction.

Regardless of the strategies used for writing drafts, the paper should be revised on the basis of whatever critical suggestions can be obtained, until it is in a clear, brief, orderly form suitable for publication. Once again, the best model for the proper final form is a good paper on a similar topic.

REVISION AFTER REVIEW BY THE JOURNAL

After the researchers have prepared the best report they can and have submitted it to a journal, they must wait for several months to get the reaction of the reviewers. In rare instances, the editor will accept the paper exactly as submitted, with no revisions required. More often, a paper will be accepted with the condition that certain specific parts be revised on the basis of the reviewers' suggestions. In some cases, the authors may be asked to resubmit a greatly revised or completely rewritten paper for a second review. Finally, the editor may inform the authors that the paper is not suitable for publication in the journal. The editor usually sends the comments of the reviewers to the authors.

Beginning writers should not be overwhelmed by critical comments of reviewers. Although the comments may seem at first to be cruel and unfair, they can be of great value. They are free advice given by experts on the topic of the research. Where the paper is accepted with minor revisions, the writers should cheerfully make revisions that do not change the meaning of the paper. For any suggestions that they do not accept, they should send a detailed statement of their reasons for rejecting the suggestion along with the revised manuscript.

Less fortunate authors who are required to make major revisions and resubmit the paper for a second review should do so when they feel that the criticisms are justified and that they are capable of making the required revisions. If they decide not to revise and resubmit, they may wish to submit the paper to another journal with different or less rigorous standards. For HCD research, however, the papers that receive the greatest attention and respect are those published in *JSHR*, *JSHD*, and other leading journals. Authors should try to swallow their pride, overcome their distaste for making yet one more revision, and do their best to put their paper into an acceptable form.

When a paper is rejected, authors may wish to submit it elsewhere, or they may accept the editor's verdict that it is not worthy of publication. It is not wise to react by abandoning the research entirely. Reviewers usually have a good perspective, and their criticisms can be used to plan research that will be accepted for publication. In cases where researchers are using a new research approach or a new technique for assessment or training, the reviewers' rejections may seem biased against innovations that go against traditional methods. There are reviewers who tenaciously guard "accepted" theories, methods, and techniques in what seems to be a narrow and dogmatic manner, and thus impede new approaches that may contribute important information. In such cases, researchers are perhaps best advised to find a journal more sympathetic to the new approach. Publication of obviously important research in other journals can lead to acceptance by the "mainstream" professional journals.

READING THE PROOF

When a paper has been accepted for publication, the authors will eventually receive a "proof" of the paper as it will appear in the journal, and will be asked to carefully read it, note any errors, and immediately return it. The authors may be tempted to scan the paper rapidly and return it, having read it carefully too many times already. However, a careful proofreading in the recommended manner (readers are referred to the APA manual) is an absolute necessity. Both small errors such as misspelled words and major errors such as omitted paragraphs or incorrectly labeled figures are easy to miss with cursory proofreading, and will come back to haunt the authors. Nothing is worse than to see an otherwise excellent paper riddled with errors, especially when they distort the findings.

PREPARING OTHER TYPES OF RESEARCH REPORTS

Written reports submitted to journals other than *JSHR* and *JSHD* may require quite different styles. Authors should use a current issue of the journal as a model for writing style. Other types of reports may be even more different, as described here.

Student Research Projects

Student research projects are usually acceptable when written in the style of *JSHR* and *JSHD*, following the guidelines of the APA manual, unless a specific style is required by the research supervisor. The main differences concern the length of sections. The introduction may be longer, with a more detailed review of previous research. More detailed descriptions of methods and results may be given, with lengthy appendices where necessary. The discussion should be long enough to demonstrate the student's understanding of the results and ability to interpret them in a creative manner. Otherwise, the student project report can closely follow the standard format. Reports of student research projects are usually considerably shorter than student theses.

Student Theses

Students should consult the regulations of their university, as well as their thesis supervisor, regarding the recommended style for master's and doctoral theses. A thesis is usually much longer than published research reports and student research projects. The sections may be divided into several chapters. Following the introduction, there is a lengthy review of the literature, sometimes divided into more than one section or chapter. Methods are described in detail, as are results. The discussion chapter must demonstrate the student's ability to understand and interpret research, and should clearly indicate the contribution to knowledge of the thesis research. A thesis on a similar topic that received a very good rating from the student's department can be used as a model.

Some universities permit students to modify the standard format by submitting research that has already been published as papers, monographs, book chapters, or books, along with a detailed review of the literature and a detailed interpretation.

Monographs

Monographs are reports of research that cannot be adequately presented within the page limits of a journal article. They often describe a series of studies rather than a single study. Thesis research may involve too much information for a single journal article, and may be published as a series of articles or a monograph. Monographs usually follow standard journal style. Authors take special care in the preparation of monographs, because they can be very substantial contributions to knowledge.

Book Chapters

Research may be reported in the form of book chapters where the findings have been presented at a conference or symposium, or where the book editor wishes to assemble a number of research reports on a particular topic. The chapter may present more than one study, and may report research plans and preliminary results of incomplete research. Research reports in book chapters may be less rigorous than research reports in journals. Authors are more free to speculate about preliminary findings. However, careless speculation not supported by later research is not a useful contribution to knowledge. Where there is no careful review of submissions, authors of book chapters must be responsible themselves for the quality of their research report.

Books

Books are very ambitious undertakings, often requiring several years for completion. Authors usually submit a preliminary outline to several publishers and sign a contract for the book before completing the final writing. Some research projects or series of studies, including student theses, merit publication in book form. Authors are more free to report the research in whatever style they wish. Publishers usually ask experts to review the final manuscript more for content than for style. Then copy editors help the author put the book in final form.

Oral Presentations

Unpublished research is often reported in oral presentations at departmental seminars and professional conferences. The style of such presentations depends on the time limitations. Where the time is limited to 10 or 15 minutes, the author should write the talk in advance and carefully rehearse it until it can be presented with proper timing and intonation.

If it is one of a series of presentations, only highlights that can be easily understood should be presented.

The problem should be briefly stated, with a very brief review of previous research. The main details of the method should be presented slowly and carefully, with appropriate audiovisual aids. Only the main details of the results that can be immediately understood by the audience should be presented. Great care should be taken with audiovisual aids to present the salient features of the findings in clear visual and audible form. Comments on audiovisual displays should be carefully rehearsed. Unrehearsed descriptions of the data in tables and figures always result in the speaker exceeding the time limit, to the great discomfort of the audience. The final conclusions should be brief and to the point.

Carefully prepared and rehearsed presentations are a credit to the speaker and to the institution they represent, and are well worth the time and effort expended in preparation. These recommendations apply equally to presentations at oral defenses of theses, which are usually about 15 to 20 minutes long.

Presentations longer than 20 minutes may be written out in advance, or presented more informally, depending on the speaker's preference. Beginning researchers may need to make formal presentations. However, there is a danger of losing the attention of the audience if the talk is read in an uninflected voice and gives details of interest only to the speaker. Once again, the more practice the better. The speaker should consciously attempt to develop effective strategies for lengthy research presentations. Less gifted speakers may take years to develop an effective style.

WORD PROCESSORS

Word processors are invaluable for the preparation of research reports. The separate sections of the reports can be kept in separate files. References can be added and deleted as needed. Where graphical presentations are important, special programs are available. Revisions of drafts and revisions of the final manuscript in response to reviewers' comments are easily done. Every aspect of writing is immeasurably facilitated.

ADDITIONAL INFORMATION

Most books on research methods contain guidelines for writing research reports. Becker (1986) has written a book for scientists about writing books, articles, and theses. Long, Convey, and Chwalek (1985) have written a systematic guide for writing dissertations in the social and behavioral sciences. Tufte (1983) has provided detailed information about the preparation of graphs.

APPENDIX
D

Answers to Exercises

CHAPTER 4

1. a. Subject controls: age, sex, linguistic background, vocabulary knowledge
      Situation controls: listening conditions, instructions, task
   b. Failure to control age, sex, linguistic background, or vocabulary knowledge
   c. Independent — speech production (articulation) disorders
      Dependent — performance on speech perception test
   d. Articulation disorder, no articulation disorder
   e. Internal validity — relevant subject and situation variables are controlled
      External validity — performance on speech perception test reflects speech perception abilities in real-life situations.
   f. Repeat test, compare scores on halves of test, compare scores on alternate forms of test
   g. No — with a pointing response, observer reliability is not a problem
2. a. Independent — training
      Dependent — fluency on speech samples

b. Before training and after training
c. Relation of fluency on speech sample to fluency in natural communicative situations
d. Assess observer reliability by determining percentage of agreement of two observers in judging fluency on speech samples
3. a. Independent — training
   Dependent — fluency on speech samples
   b. Training, no training
   c. Age, sex, education, severity of stuttering, history of treatment; instructions, method of recording speech sample, training procedure
   d. The untrained group
   e. Failure to match groups in severity of stuttering

CHAPTER 5

1. One independent variable, two levels of independent variable, one dependent variable
2. The desirable minimum is 20 (10 per group) and the absolute minimum is 10 (5 per group)
3. (1) natural group, (2) repeated measurement, (3) matched group
4. Personality problems: combined matched and natural group
   Speech aid: repeated measurement or matched group
   Speech discrimination tests: repeated measurement
5. Independent variable — hearing aids
   Levels of the independent variable — standard and new hearing aids
   Dependent variable — a measure of hearing (e.g., pure tone test)
   Relevant controls — age, sex, amount and type of hearing loss; listening situation, hearing test
   Random assignment design: randomly assign subjects to two groups from available population of hearing impaired; test one aid with each group
   Matched group design: match two groups from available population of hearing impaired in age, sex, amount and type of hearing loss; test one aid with each group
   Repeated measurement design: select a representative group of hearing impaired from available population; test both aids with the entire group; counterbalance order of presentation of aids by testing half of the subjects with one aid first and the other half with the other aid first

CHAPTER 6

1. a. 2×2 repeated measures factorial design
      Independent — background noise (quiet and noise), word context (isolated words, words in sentences)
      Dependent — performance on word recognition test
      Minimum subjects — 20 to 40
      Order of presentation of background noise and of word context must be counterbalanced
      Example of interaction — the effects of noise as compared with quiet are greater for words in isolation than words in sentences
   b. Independent group design with more than two levels
      Independent — age (age 1, age 2, age 3, etc.)
      Dependent — performance on speech perception test
      Minimum subjects — 5 to 10 per level
      No counterbalancing or interaction
   c. 2×2 independent group design
      Independent — voice disorder (voice disorder, no voice disorder), sex
      Dependent — judgment of speech intelligibility from speech sample
      Minimum subjects — 20 to 40
      No counterbalancing required
      Example of interaction — the difference between normal and voice-disordered female subjects is smaller than the difference between male subjects
   d. Repeated measurement design with more than two levels
      Independent — background noise (quiet, low noise, moderate noise, etc.)
      Dependent — performance on speech perception tests
      Minimum subjects — 5 to 10 per level
      Counterbalance order of background noise
      No interaction
   e. 2×2 mixed factorial design
      Independent — voice disorder (voice disorder, no voice disorder), phoneme class (vowels, consonants)
      Dependent — judged intelligibility of vowels and consonants in a standardized speech sample
      Minimum subjects — 20 to 40
      No counterbalancing necessary (vowels and consonants evenly distributed in speech sample)
      Example of interaction — difference between voice disorder and no voice disorder groups is greatest for vowels

CHAPTER 13

1. a. MAIN EFFECTS: Hearing Aids (Aid 1, Aid 2)
                        Noise (Quiet, Noise)
    INTERACTION: Hearing Aids × Noise

   b. MAIN EFFECTS: Age (young, older)
                        Sex (girls, boys)
                        Task (picture description, story retelling)
    INTERACTIONS: Age × Sex
                        Age × Task
                        Sex × Task
                        Age × Sex × Task

   c. MAIN EFFECTS: Age (young, older)
                        Education (high school, university)
                        Amount of Training (0 weeks, 4 weeks, 8 weeks)
                        Amount of Hearing Loss (Moderate, Severe)
    INTERACTIONS: Age × Education
                        Age × Training
                        Age × Hearing
                        Education × Training
                        Education × Hearing
                        Training × Hearing
                        Age × Education × Training
                        Age × Education × Hearing
                        Age × Training × Hearing
                        Education × Training × Hearing
                        Age × Education × Training × Hearing

2. a. There is better speech discrimination with Hearing Aid 1 in quiet, and with Hearing Aid 2 in noise

   b. Younger boys, older boys, and older girls make more errors in story retelling than in picture description. Older girls make the same amount of errors in story retelling and picture description

   c. All groups show continued improvement with training from 4 weeks to 8 weeks except the younger university educated group with moderate hearing loss, who reach maximum performance in 4 weeks

(Note: The easiest examples of higher-order interactions are those where one cell shows a different trend for a main effect, as illustrated by the example of a 2×2×2 interaction in the text.)

REFERENCES

Aanstoos, C. M. (1987). A comparative survey of human science psychologies. *Methods*, *1*(2), 1–37.

Anastasi, A. (1982). *Psychological testing* (5th ed.). New York: Macmillan.

Barker, H. R., & Barker, B. M. (1984). *Multivariate analysis of variance*. University, AL: University of Alabama Press.

Barlow, D. H., Hayes, S. C., & Nelson, R .O. (1984). *The scientist practitioner*. Elmsford, NY: Pergamon Press.

Barlow, D. H., & Herson, M. (1984). *Single case experimental designs*. Elmsford, NY: Pergamon Press.

Becker, H. S. (1986). *Writing for social scientists: How to start and finish your thesis, book, or article*. Chicago: University of Chicago Press.

Borchardt, D. H., & Francis, R. D. (1984). *How to find out in psychology: A guide to literature and methods of research*. Elmsford, NY: Pergamon Press.

Bray, J. H., & Maxwell, S. E. (1985). *Multivariate analysis of variance*. Beverly Hills, CA: Sage.

Brewer, M. B., & Collins, B. E. (Eds.) (1981). *Scientific inquiry and the social sciences: A volume in honor of Donald T. Campbell*. San Francisco: Jossey-Bass.

Bromley, D. B. (1986). *The case-study method in psychology and related disciplines*. Chichester, England: John Wiley.

Bruning, J. L., & Kintz, B. L. (1987). *Computational handbook of statistics* (3rd ed.). Glenview, IL: Scott, Foresman.

Calfee, R. C. (1985). *Experimental methods in psychology*. New York: Holt, Rinehart & Winston.

Cherulnik, P. D. (1983). *Behavioral research*. New York: Harper & Row.

Clayton, K. N. (1984). *An introduction to statistics*. Columbus, OH: Charles E. Merrill.

Cochran, W. G., Moses, L. E., & Mosteller, F. (1983). *Planning and analysis of observational studies*. New York: Wiley.

Connell, P. J., & Thompson, C.K. (1986). Flexibility of single-subject experimental designs. Part III: Using flexibility to design or modify experiments. *Journal of Speech and Hearing Disorders, 51,* 214–225.

Cook, T. D., & Campbell, D. T. (1979). *Quasi-experimentation: Design and analysis issues for field settings.* Boston, MA: Houghton Mifflin.

Crano, W. D., & Brewer, M. B. (1986). *Principles and methods of social research.* Boston: Allyn & Bacon.

Cureton, E. E., & D'Agostino, R. B. (1983). *Factor analysis.* Hillsdale, NJ: Erlbaum.

Edwards, A. L. (1984). *An introduction to linear regression and correlation* (2nd ed.). New York: Freeman.

Edwards, A. L. (1985). *Experimental design in psychological research* (5th ed.). New York: Harper & Row.

Elman, J. L., & McLelland, J. L. (1984). Speech perception as a cognitive process. In N. J. Lass (Ed.), *Speech and language: Advances in basic research and practice* (Vol. 10). New York: Academic Press.

Elmes, D. G., Kantowitz, B. H., & Roediger, H. L. (1985). *Research methods in psychology* (2nd ed.). St. Paul, MN: West.

Fallik, F., & Brown, B. (1983). *Statistics for behavioral sciences.* Homewood, IL: Dorsey Press.

Fiske, D. W., & Schweder, R. A. (Eds.) (1986). *Metatheory in social science: Pluralism and subjectives.* Chicago: University of Chicago Press.

Fodor, J. A. (1983). *The modularity of mind.* Cambridge, MA: MIT Press.

Fowler, F. J. (1984). *Survey research methods.* Beverly Hills, CA: Sage.

Friedman, M. (1984). *Contemporary psychology.* Pittsburgh, PA: Duquesne University Press.

Giorgi, A. (1985). *Phenomenology and psychological research.* Pittsburgh, PA: Duquesne University Press.

Goetz, J. P., & LeCompte, M. D. (1984). *Ethnography and quantitative design in educational research.* New York: Academic Press.

Gorsuch, R. L. (1983). *Factor analysis* (2nd ed.). Hillsdale, NJ: Erlbaum.

Hardcastle, W. J., Barry, R. A. M., & Clark, C. J. (1987). An instrumental phonetic study of lingual activity in articulation-disordered children. *Journal of Speech and Hearing Research, 30,* 171–184.

Hartmann, D. P. (1982). *Using observers to study behavior.* San Francisco: Jossey-Bass.

Hays, W. L. (1981). *Statistics* (3rd ed.). New York: Holt, Rinehart & Winston.

Hegde, M. N. (1987). *Clinical research in communicative disorders.* San Diego: College-Hill Press/Little, Brown.

Howard, G. S. (1985). *Basic research methods in the social sciences.* Glenview, IL: Scott, Foresman.

Kearns, K. P. (1986). Flexibility of single-subject experimental designs. Part II: Design selection and arrangement in experimental phases. *Journal of Speech and Hearing Disorders, 51,* 204–213.

Keppel, G. (1982). *Design and analysis* (2nd ed.). Englewood Cliffs, NJ: Prentice-Hall.

Kirk, R. E. (1984). *Elementary statistics* (2nd ed.). Monterey, CA: Brooks/Cole.

Kratochwill, T. R. (1978). *Single-subject research.* New York: Academic Press.

Light, L., & Pillemer, D. B. (1984). *The science of reviewing research.* Cambridge, MA: Harvard University Press.

Liles, B. Z. (1987). Episode organization and cohesive conjunctives in narratives of children with and without language disorders. *Journal of Speech and Hearing Research, 30,* 185–196.

Lofland, J., & Lofland, L. H. (1984). *Analyzing social settings: A guide to qualitative observation and analysis.* Belmont, CA: Wadsworth.

Long, T. J., Convey, J. J., & Chwalek, A. R. (1985). *Completing dissertations in the behavioral sciences and education.* San Francisco: Jossey-Bass.

Lorr, M. (1983). *Cluster analysis for social scientists.* San Francisco: Jossey-Bass.

Ludlow, C. L., & Connor, N. P. (1987). Dynamic aspects of phonatory control in spasmodic dysphonia. *Journal of Speech and Hearing Research, 30,* 197–206.

Marcus, G. E., & Fischer, M. M. (1986). *Anthropology as cultural critique.* Chicago, IL: University of Chicago Press.

Martin, D. W. (1985). *Doing psychology experiments.* Monterey, CA: Brooks/Cole.

McReynolds, L. J., & Kearns, K. P. (1983). *Single-subject experimental designs in communicative disorders.* Baltimore, MD: University Park Press.

McReynolds, L. J., & Thompson, C.K. (1986). Flexibility of single-subject experimental designs. Part I: Review of the basics of single-subject designs. *Journal of Speech and Hearing Disorders, 51,* 194–203.

Pedhazur, E., & Kerlinger, F. N. (1982). *Multiple regression in behavioral research* (2nd ed.). New York: Holt, Rinehart & Winston.

Penner, M. J. (1987). Masking of tinnitus and central masking. *Journal of Speech and Hearing Research, 30,* 147–152.

Pickering, M. (1984). Interpersonal communication in speech-language supervisory conferences: A qualitative study. *Journal of Speech and Hearing Disorders, 49,* 189–195.

Polkinghorne, D. (1983). *Methodology for the human sciences.* Albany, NY: State University of New York Press.

Quarles, S. D. (1986). *Guide to federal funding for social scientists.* NY: Russell Sage Foundation.

Ray, W. J., & Ravizza, R. (1985). *Methods toward a science of behavior and experience* (2nd ed.). Belmont, CA: Wadsworth.

Rubenstein, A., & Boothroyd, A. (1987). Effect of two approaches to auditory training on speech recognition by hearing-impaired adults. *Journal of Speech and Hearing Research, 30,* 153–160.

Rumelhart, D. E., & McClelland, J. L. (1986). *Parallel distributed processing.* Cambridge, MA: MIT Press.

Shaughnessy, J. J., & Zechmeister, E. B. (1985). *Research methods in psychology.* New York: Alfred A. Knopf.

Shearer, W. M. (1982). *Research processes in speech, language, and hearing.* Baltimore: Williams & Wilkins.

Siegel, S. (1956). *Nonparametric statistics for the behavioral sciences.* New York: McGraw-Hill.

Silverman, F. H. (1977). *Research design in speech pathology and audiology.* Englewood Cliffs, NJ: Prentice-Hall.

Smith, R. V. (1984). *Graduate research: A guide for students in the sciences*. Philadelphia: ISI Press.

Solso, R. L., & Johnson, H. H. (1984). *An introduction to experimental design in psychology: A case approach* (3rd ed.). New York: Harper & Row.

Sommer, R., & Sommer, B. B. (1986). *A practical guide to behavioral research: Tools and techniques* (2nd ed.). New York: Oxford University Press.

Spence, J. T., Cotton, J. W., Underwood, B. J. & Duncan, C. P. (1983). *Elementary statistics* (4th ed.). Englewood Cliffs, NJ: Prentice-Hall.

Spradley, J. P. (1979). *The ethnographic interview*. New York: Holt, Rinehart & Winston.

Tabachnick, B. G., & Fidell, L. S. (1983). *Using multivariate statistics*. New York: Harper & Row.

Tawney, J. W., & Gast, D. L. (1984). *Single subject research in special education*. Columbus, OH: Charles E. Merrill.

Taylor, S. J., & Bogdan, R. (1984). *Introduction to qualitative research methods*. New York: Wiley.

Tufte, E. R. (1983). *The visual display of quantitative information*. Cheshire, CT: Graphics Press.

Ventry, I. M., & Schiavetti, N. (1980). *Evaluating research in speech pathology and audiology*. New York: John Wiley & Sons.

Wiley, T. L., Oviatt, D. L., & Block, M. G. (1987). Acoustic-immitance measures in normal ears. *Journal of Speech and Hearing Research, 30*, 161–170.

Yaremko, R. M., Harari, H., Harrison, R. C., & Lynn, E. (1986). *Handbook of research and quantitative methods in psychology*. Hillsdale, NJ: Erlbaum.

SUBJECT INDEX

Notes

Notes

Notes

Notes

Notes

Notes

Notes

Notes

Notes

Notes